PRIMARY CARE

STATE OF HEALTH SERIES

Edited by Chris Ham, Director of Health Services Management Centre, University of Birmingham

PRIMARY CARE
Making connections

Noel Boaden

Open University Press
Buckingham · Philadelphia

Open University Press
Celtic Court
22 Ballmoor
Buckingham
MK18 1XW

and
1900 Frost Road, Suite 101
Bristol, PA 19007, USA

First Published 1997

A catalogue record of this book is available from the British Library

ISBN   0 335 197485 (pb)   0 335 197493 (hb)

Library of Congress Cataloging-in-Publication Data
Boaden, Noel.
    Primary care : making connections / Noel Boaden.
        p.   cm.—(State of health series)
    Includes bibliographical references and index.
    ISBN   0-335-19749-3 (hardcover).—ISBN   0-335-19748-5 (pbk.)
    1. Primary health care—Great Britain—Administration.
2. National Health Services (Great Britain)—Administration.
I. Title. II. Series.
    [DNLM: 1. Primary Health Care—organization & administration—
Great Britain.   2. National Health Programs—organization &
administration—Great Britain.   W 84.6 B662p 1997]
RA427.9.B63   1997
362.1'0941—dc21
DNLM/DLC
for Library of Congress   97-13905
                                                                                CIP

Typeset by Type Study, Scarborough
Printed in Great Britain by St Edmundsbury Press,
Bury St Edmunds, Suffolk

CONTENTS

ACKNOWLEDGEMENTS

I am grateful to a number of people for help and support in the writing of this book. Professor John Bligh first involved me in debate about quality in general practice some five years ago and has been a constant support since that time. His Department of Health Care Education at the University of Liverpool has provided me with a base and valued support during the last year. Dr Tony Mathie enabled me to become involved in the education of general practitioners and he and his colleagues involved in professional education, especially the GP Tutors in the Mersey Region, have provided much stimulating opportunity for me to discuss ideas about general practice and primary care. Astra Pharmaceuticals kindly provided financial support during the preparation of the book. Finally and most significantly my thanks are due to my wife Margaret who has been a stimulus and a sounding board and has helped shape my ideas about primary care over a number of years while bearing with the domestic failings which writing seems to produce.

SERIES EDITOR'S INTRODUCTION

Health services in many developed countries have come under critical scrutiny in recent years. In part this is because of increasing expenditure, much of it funded from public sources, and the pressure this has put on governments seeking to control public spending. Also important has been the perception that resources allocated to health services are not always deployed in an optimal fashion. Thus at a time when the scope for increasing expenditure is extremely limited, there is a need to search for ways of using existing budgets more efficiently. A further concern has been the desire to ensure access to health care of various groups on an equitable basis. In some countries this has been linked to a wish to enhance patient choice and to make service providers more responsive to patients as 'consumers'.

Underlying these specific concerns are a number of more fundamental developments which have a significant bearing on the performance of health services. Three are worth highlighting. First, there are demographic changes, including the ageing population and the decline in the proportion of the population of working age. These changes will both increase the demand for health care and at the same time limit the ability of health services to respond to this demand.

Second, advances in medical science will also give rise to new demands within the health services. These advances cover a range of possibilities, including innovations in surgery, drug therapy, screening and diagnosis. The pace of innovation is likely to quicken as the end of the century approaches, with significant implications for the funding and provision of services.

Third, public expectations of health services are rising as those who use services demand higher standards of care. In part, this is stimulated by developments within the health service, including the availability of new technology. More fundamentally, it stems from the emergence of a more educated and informed population, in which people are accustomed to being treated as consumers rather than patients.

Against this background, policymakers in a number of countries are reviewing the future of health services. Those countries which have traditionally relied on a market in health care are making greater use of regulation and planning. Equally, those countries which have traditionally relied on regulation and planning are moving towards a more competitive approach. In no country is there complete satisfaction with existing methods of financing and delivery, and everywhere there is a search for new policy instruments.

The aim of this series is to contribute to debate about the future of health services through an analysis of major issues in health policy. These issues have been chosen because they are both of current interest and of enduring importance. The series is intended to be accessible to students and informed lay readers as well as to specialists working in this field. The aim is to go beyond a textbook approach to health policy analysis and to encourage authors to move debate about their issue forward. In this sense, each book presents a summary of current research and thinking, and an exploration of future policy directions.

Professor Chris Ham
Director of Health Services Management Centre
University of Birmingham

ABBREVIATIONS

A and E	accident and emergency
AHA	area health authorities
CHC	Community Health Councils
FHSA	Family Health Service Authorities
GP	general practitioner
HA	health authority
NHS	National Health Service
PAMs	professions associated with medicine
PGEA	Postgraduate Education Allowance
PHCT	Primary Health Care Team
RCGP	Royal College of General Practitioners
WHO	World Health Organization

INTRODUCTION

The National Health Service (NHS) of Great Britain has been at the centre of political debate since the middle of the 1980s and has been the subject of what seems like constant reform ever since with the pace of change showing no sign of slowing. This reform process is significant because it reflects a breakdown in the long-standing political consensus about the character of the NHS with doubts even being expressed about it surviving in its traditional form. This is because the reforms have been driven by the New Conservatism which adopts a political philosophy which advocates a reduced role for the state in providing welfare, fuelled by an economic analysis which believes that economic prosperity is dependent on limiting public borrowing and state expenditure. Both views pose an implicit threat to the traditional NHS and have assumed much greater significance, and had more impact than might normally be the case, because one party has held office and determined public policy for nearly two decades. The piecemeal and incremental (or decremental) pattern of change in public policy has not itself changed, but its cumulative impact over so many years has heightened its effect on the NHS and on other related areas of public policy.

The impact of change over such a long period has been heightened by associated changes in the way in which policy is developed and introduced. Despite a philosophy advocating a reduced role for government, the reform process has involved the government in a highly directive role. The corporate, consensus-building process of the past has given way to more limited public discussion, with professional interests more marginalized in the debate, and with the unusual addition of consultation with, and the adoption of concepts from, the private sector. These changes in the policy making process have allowed more speedy decisions to be made about policy and strong majorities in Parliament have guaranteed their passage into law. The process has substantially ignored those who will have to implement the changes, and seems to assume that implementation will be straightforward, despite much evidence of failure to implement reform successfully in the past.

This is significant because the reforms have introduced radical changes in the processes of health care delivery and mark a complete break with some of the core traditions of the NHS. In the new NHS resource allocation, service delivery and quality will be determined through a quasi-market in health care. Local health organizations become either purchasers or providers (or in the case of some general practices, both) within the quasi-market. Organizationally, stressing improved management reflects a push towards greater emphasis being placed on efficiency within the new NHS, and also a wish to overcome the perceived professional dominance of the traditional approach. These changes are driven by a belief that markets are the most efficient way to allocate resources, and a perception that traditional public sector allocations have often worked in the interests of those providing services within the NHS, rather than of the patients being treated. An effective market, and competent management will allow expenditure to be cut, but service standards maintained, through improved efficiency and the removal of 'restrictive working practices'. This has involved reorganizing structures, changing patterns of public spending and directly challenging the role, autonomy and power of the professions within the system. Taken together these changes constitute a coherent and radical reform of the NHS.

The style of the policy process, and the substance of the policy have changed the balance of debate. They have increased the significance of the local levels of decision making and their role in the process of converting broad central policy change into reformed practice on the ground. Traditionally the professional and political interests would have been consulted and expected to raise the problems of implementation during the policy debate. This often had a conservative influence on possible reforms with the interests of current providers successfully preventing major changes in policy, often by invoking difficulties of implementation. Limiting consultation with them does not alter the fact that current service providers remain vital in the process of implementing change. Non-consultation of their interests, real or perceived, may lead to mistakes in policy making, difficulties at the implementation stage and may even result in only part, or even non-compliance with new practice. Such possibilities are more likely in a complex, large-scale service like the NHS, with a fragmented structure and high levels of professional autonomy coupled with an historical record of more modest reform. Service delivery in health care gives great autonomy to professional judgement and decision making, causing core service activity to become inherently difficult to control and making implementation of reform a complex process. Indeed, the Conservative government through the NHS Executive, repeatedly make the point that their role is to create a framework leaving responsibility for implementation within that framework to reflect local needs and priorities. At the same time there is a constant flow of central direction, guidance and advice about local practice.

PRIMARY CARE

The impact of changing process and policy is evident in the importance placed on the clear intention to give 'primary care' a leading role in the future development of the NHS. The emphasis on primary care has been seen as serving the wider agenda, changing the balance of power within the medical profession, shifting the focus of health care activity away from the hospitals, and most importantly reducing the escalating cost of health care. This has been implicit in the detailed policies such as care in the community introduced in 1990, and in the proposed reorganization of medical care in London following the Tomlinson Report of 1992, and has been explicit in detailed changes in primary care itself.

Given the new 'politics of reform' it is not surprising that this has evoked a mixed response from those involved in primary care. Early in the process the Royal College of General Practitioners (RCGP) welcomed 'the clear recognition of the central importance of general practice by Government' when responding to the Conservative government's Agenda for Discussion (RCGP 1987). The warmth of that general welcome from the profession for a 'primary care led NHS' has been in marked contrast to the much cooler response to particular changes proposed by the government as being essential to its implementation. There was conflict in 1990 during the debate about the introduction of a new GP contract, which marked the first direct intervention by government into the clinical practice of GPs. Fundholding by general practices, introduced only a year after the contract, but seen by the government as central to the new market and to strengthening the hand of general practice in relation to secondary care, has been equally controversial. Professional opinion is sharply divided about the utility and impact of fundholding but this has not prevented a steady expansion of the scheme to involve purchasing of all aspects of care and to cover more than half of the British population. These controversies, about the specifics and the speed of change, are reflected at a more general level in a reported loss of morale among GPs, and consequent problems in retaining doctors in primary care, and recruiting their successors.

None of this is surprising. In part the ambiguous response results from the distinction between the generalities of broad policy and the hard realities of detailed implementation. The lack of clarity in the broad debate often allows those involved, and those affected but not involved, to interpret proposals in line with their own wishes and interests. Implementation, when it comes, removes that luxury. It requires clarity on all sides and gives substance to the meanings which were obscured in the more general discussion. This is true of all public service policy but is particularly relevant in primary care.

The response also reflects a lack of clarity about what constitutes primary care. General practice has until recently been synonymous with primary care in much of the debate within the NHS. This view is now accepted as being too narrow, even by the RCGP. The widening scope of primary care is most evident in discussion about the Primary Health Care Team (PHCT) and about consequent multi-professional education and training for its members. Development of such teams reflects the problem of implementing reform around this wider notion of primary care. The range of potential members of a PHCT remains a matter of debate. Accepted core members (GP, practice nurse, district nurse and health visitor) are now more likely to be found working from the same health centre, or from within the same general practice. Which other professions, and which associated staff should also join the team, is less clear and practice remains highly varied. Whether any extended PHCTs exist, and how they organize and manage their work, is not clear but it seems probable that few are yet functioning fully as operational teams. Certainly the scope and scale of general practice remains very diverse, though fundholding has created opportunities for widening the membership of the PHCT.

This is but one of the uncertainties in the reformed situation. Despite this, there is recognition of the need for change in the range of services which are offered in primary care, how their delivery is organized and who will be the key professions involved. It is also recognized that this will change relationships within primary care and those between primary and secondary care. The implications for contact with agencies in related social service fields are less clear but are seen to be on the agenda, if only because they hold budgets for care in the community provision. Uncertainty around all these issues is reinforced by a lack of clarity about what is meant by a leading role for primary care within the NHS.

Despite such uncertainties some GPs have begun to adopt the reforms and adapt their practice, most obviously GP fundholders, particularly those involved in total fundholding. Others have rejected fundholding but taken a different route adopting other models of purchasing for secondary care. This reflects the diverse pattern of innovation in general practice discussed by Leese and Bosanquet (1995a, 1995b). The broad mixture of opposition, uncertainty, acceptance and keen adoption is typical of the range of responses to change in the NHS and also needs to be seen against the development of primary care within the NHS (Stocking 1985). Reform and reorganization have taken place at regular intervals in the organization of secondary and community care within the NHS though with less impact than was hoped for on patterns of work and the distribution of influence over policy and resource allocation. Primary care, or more accurately general practice, has been much more resistant to change. Having secured contractual independence for GPs at the creation of the NHS, the profession has always fought to maintain that formal position and with it a high degree of autonomy and control over the organization and character of practice. General reform has been on the government agenda at various times but has not happened, partly because of professional opposition and of cost. There have been developments like the creation of health centres and of larger group partnerships, but these have been the product of individual decisions by doctors, albeit helped by general financial arrangements. The development of vocational training for general practice has been a major general change, but the core activity of general practice has remained largely the same and a broader model of integrated primary care has not developed very far.

This history makes the recent reforms, widely perceived as being imposed on, and not negotiated with the profession, particularly difficult for doctors. The reforms challenge both their traditional professional autonomy as practitioners, and their collective dominance of decision making about the organization and delivery of care. Whether government or profession is right about how to organize primary care, and how current performance should be judged, is another matter. The traditional model of family medicine has been strained by the mounting demand for treatment and the failure to adapt organization and practice more fundamentally to cope with that strain. The length of consultations remains too short for best practice, prescribing remains extensive and the pressures felt by doctors reflect a profession struggling to maintain its traditions rather than one adjusting creatively to change. Most importantly, inequalities in the health status and access to health care of the population remain substantial, associated with wide variations in the availability, practice and quality of primary care (Townsend *et al.* 1988).

The blame does not rest entirely with primary care. Attempts have been made periodically to shift the balance of care between sectors, but have always foundered on the rock of established medical politics and the complex divisions within the NHS and between the NHS and local government. Most significantly resource limitations have always inhibited what could be achieved. Redistribution of money from secondary care has not proved easy, and extra resources to lubricate the process of change have seldom been forthcoming. Significantly the argument seems to have been between politicians seeking a shift towards primary care and community care, with hospital consultants successfully defending their sector. General practice has defended its traditional autonomy but has failed to secure the resources needed for serious development of primary care. Current reactions suggest that may reflect some ambiguity about the role of primary care within the NHS.

All of this has now changed. Driven in the main by the escalating costs of hospital care the politics of recent reform have changed the structure of secondary care and the relationship between sectors, requiring complementary changes in primary care. Those changes have still to materialize and there is evidence that changes in practice are not yet as far reaching as the policy intended or as the adoption of formal structures might suggest (Audit Commission 1996b).

THE NEED FOR FURTHER REFORM

Achievement of the goal of a primary-led NHS will, it is clear, require more than the formal changes already announced, and the relocation of health and related work into the community. It will require new structures and forms of organization within primary health care and within related services, some of which are already beginning to appear as a result of local initiatives (Meads 1996). It will involve more resources being spent within the community, not only on health care, but on a more broadly defined primary care. More importantly, if it is to have impact on those in need of care, it will require widespread changes in the attitudes and values, and the approach to their work, of everyone working in health care, and in particular those involved in primary care.

Structural change is important, but it may need to be more radical in primary care than the present reforms. Creation of a suitable environment for PHCTs to develop will require a wider look at new forms of organization, not merely at voluntary adaptations of general practice. Interprofessional working, which goes beyond the multiprofessional ideas already being introduced in some areas, requires radical changes in decision making about care and appropriate resource allocation. Improved accountability in any new arrangements will need to take into account the rights of patients as well as those of professional staff involved.

Structural change by itself will not be enough however. Operation of any new structures will require changes in professional attitudes, values and practice if it is to succeed. This change in the culture of primary care will require changes in professional education and training and in the traditional concept of the professional career. The exclusivity of the traditional professional model, successfully achieved by medicine, and sought after by associated professions, is a poor model for the team work inherent in the new primary care. Years of initial training for a lengthy career are ill-suited to the adaptability and flexibility which will be required in the new system, and which are manifestly missing among those failing to cope with the current changes in primary care. Undergraduate education will need to change, and is beginning to do so. Postgraduate training will need to follow suit and most importantly, continuing professional development will need to become as important as early professional training.

The organization and content of professional education will also need to change to reflect changing patterns of service and consequent changes in the relationships and patterns of power and influence experienced in primary care. Needs assessment, resource allocation, health advocacy, and the managerial skills needed to bring them together without detriment to the best of existing care will demand far-reaching changes.

THE PLAN OF THE BOOK

This book seeks to address these issues. It is concerned with the changes in structure and culture which will be needed if a primary-led NHS is to be achieved. Throughout it will be concerned to explore both the narrow view of primary care as little more than general practice, and the extended view which embraces a much wider spectrum of activity. This involves consideration of the core professions of general practice, community nursing and social work. The implications for other associated professions are not considered although it is hoped that the arguments may readily be extended to them by those involved.

The first two chapters recognize the need to understand the historical background out of which the present situation has emerged. Chapter 1 charts the evolution of public services and in particular of health services from their origins in the nineteenth century through to 1980. Chapter 2 takes up that profile of development and examines the very active reforms which have been introduced since 1984 and which provide the detailed framework within which the new primary care is to be delivered. Chapter 3 builds on this background and examines what is meant by primary care, how that affects who should be involved in the new primary care and goes on to examine the current position in so far as data allow. This chapter also looks at the criteria by which the new primary care should be judged.

Against this background the development of a primary care-led NHS suggests the need for further reform. Chapter 4 suggests that a systems approach might provide a useful basis from which to consider both the history of development and the issues which should inform future reform in primary care. Chapters 5 and 6 examine two central issues that arise from this approach. The first concerns the culture of primary care as it manifests itself in the professional staff involved. It examines the nature of professionalism, looks at the professional roles involved in primary care and considers the shape and character of future professional careers. Chapter 6 examines the current structure of the NHS and the organization and management of primary care and highlights the needs which are raised in relation to the intentions of reform.

The next three chapters examine proposals for reform. Chapter 7 looks at current efforts to engage with continuing professional development in primary care and concludes with proposals about how professional education might develop for the new primary care. Chapter 8 in turn looks at some of the efforts being made to engage reform within the current structures and makes proposals for more far-reaching organizational change to facilitate development. Chapter 9 recognizes the political sensitivity of all these changes and the need within the NHS to engage with political processes at a variety of levels. This chapter considers the issues which arise in relation to the formal politics of NHS decision making and the relationship between the levels of decision, central and local. It also looks at the wider issue of the relationship of health care to the people, both as patients and as citizens who pay for and use the service. A final chapter summarizes the debate and points the way to possible ways forward in the context of the most recent Conservative government proposals for further development.

HEALTH AND HEALTH CARE IN SOCIETY: MISSING LINKS

Every health services system has two main goals. The first is to optimize the health of the population by employing the most advanced knowledge about the causation of disease, illness management, and health maximization. The second, and equally important, goal is to minimize the disparities across population sub-groups to ensure equal access to health services and the ability to achieve optimal health.

(Starfield 1992: 3)

There would be little disagreement that optimal health for all is the prime goal of the NHS, nor that equal access to health care is a major condition for its achievement. There would be disagreement, however, about what is meant by optimal health and by equal access. There would be disagreement about the causes of ill-health and about how they might best be tackled. There would be disagreement over the management of illness when it did arise, and over the best way to achieve equal access, both to services and to health. Evidence about the health of the nation, about patterns of health care and about access to that health care, confirms the impact of such disagreement, but also shows that progress has been made towards both of Starfield's goals (Townsend *et al.* 1988). Several factors help to explain the slowness of progress and the failures that have occurred despite the creation of an advanced health care system and substantial public expenditure on care.

One explanation is lack of agreement about what constitutes health and, by inference, optimal health. There is the long established idea of health as the absence of disease, an idea that has promoted treatment as the core function of the health service and fostered the 'medical model' as the basis of that treatment. Another view broadens that definition to embrace a more comprehensive notion of health that relates not only to disease in the medical sense, but is a reflection of how individuals function within their wider social context. This broader view reaches its widest form in the World Health Organization (WHO) definition of health as a 'state of complete physical, mental and social well being and not merely the absence of disease or infirmity' (cited in Allsop 1984).

Inevitably the adoption and interpretation of these definitions differs widely across cultures, across social groups and across generations. They will also vary according to one's role and position in society and, most significantly within the health care system. The individual's view of health depends on his or her own experience, expectations and place in society. Politicians involved in deciding policy about health care will take varying views depending on their different ideologies, constituencies and the political costs and consequences of implementing their views. Professionals within the health care system will be motivated by different concerns but will also differ in their views. The consultant surgeon may take a narrow 'medical' view when treating a patient, while the GP, community nurse or social worker may work within a broader view of health. The WHO ideal extends beyond the usual scope of any of the professional or political groups within the system so that its achievement would pose a fundamental challenge to existing structures and relationships.

A second explanation lies in the complex range of factors which affect the incidence of disease and illness and consequently the attainment of physical and social well-being. Good health, and indeed ill-health, depend on the mix of economic, social and environmental conditions in which people live, and these vary widely both between and within countries, at the broad regional level, and also within quite small geographical areas. For example, poor standards of housing can directly cause disease, but they can also generate stress within families and neighbourhoods which gives rise to ill-health. Better quality housing at much greater cost, especially where income is not adequate to the rent level or the cost of purchase and maintenance, can stretch family budgets and generate considerable stress. The medical model has generated treatment for the diseases caused by bad housing. The wider social model has prompted changes in the housing system to remove the underlying causes of stress. The WHO model would involve both of these approaches reinforced by consideration of employment, income level and other sources of assistance to remedy the situation.

A third explanation involves the way in which services are delivered and their relative accessibility to different people. Before the advent of a state health care system, private and charitable services were available, but popular access to them was limited by their scale, the cost of private care, and by the tests of eligibility applied when provision of charitable care was being decided. This gave rise to highly unequal health care, invariably reinforcing the basic inequalities in health, and was one of the triggers which led to the introduction of a state system of health care. The creation of such a system did not, however, provide an automatic solution to the problem of differential access. Rather it revealed several influences on access. One was the extensive need for health care, hidden by the absence of information about the state of the people's health and the limited availability of care. Another was that the creation of a state system started a revolution of rising expectations and promoted greater demand for care. The third was that action to meet such need was limited by the capacity of medicine to provide treatment and by our collective willingness to tax and spend on providing health care.

The corollary has always been, and continues to be, a need to ration access to care even where it is ostensibly freely available. The system of rationing adopted dictates the pattern of access but the essential character of health care services makes it difficult to secure an equitable distribution. Diagnosis of disease and decisions about any resulting treatment are both determined by professionals within the system, with the patient enjoying only limited capacity to determine what should be done. Determination of the level of need for care results from the decisions of thousands of professional and non-professional carers and gatekeepers whose decisions in turn condition our ideas about our so-called rights to receive care. Carers' and gatekeepers' decisions reflect their views about health and about appropriate care, as well as being conditioned by who is seeking help and by the availability of resources to provide care. In turn, experience of this process has an effect on those seeking care, who may perceive their need, but who have to negotiate effective demand for service with professional staff. Refusal by a doctor of care to a smoker is a modern example of this process. Another is the presentation of medical symptoms because they legitimize access to medical care even though the underlying problem is often not medical.

THE BEGINNINGS OF PUBLIC HEALTH CARE

These issues can be seen operating throughout the development of health and related services in Britain. The nineteenth century offers clear illustration of their effect (Fraser 1973). Rapid population growth concentrated in urban areas, together with associated industrialization had serious effects on the health of the people. Their impact was more severe because existing private provision had neither the capacity nor the motivation to deal with the effects and a public system to do so had not yet emerged. The results were manifest in appalling living conditions for many with high consequent rates of mortality and frequent epidemics of cholera and other diseases. The health care system, such as it was, catered for the affluent but could not protect them from the impact of infectious diseases. Such diseases were not selective in their impact and escape from the city into suburbia or the countryside was not feasible for most people. The search for alternative strategies resulted in the public health movement of the mid-nineteenth century. Doctors were among the main advocates of action. The scope of medicine itself in treating disease was limited but the cause of some diseases was understood and they could be tackled at source. The result was new drains, sewers and water supply, 'public goods' which at once affected whole localities with significant gains in health status and some equality of access to the benefits which flow from such public services.

At the same time other factors that benefit the public health were beginning to be the subject of government action. Though not motivated directly by concern for health, education came early onto the agenda. Voluntary schools received public funding from 1836, and the state moved into direct provision after 1870, introducing compulsory attendance and slowly raising the school leaving age thereafter. Housing was different in that it was recognized as a direct health issue motivating the introduction of state control over the quality of housing conditions, though producing only token efforts to provide public housing at this time. Minimal effort was made to deal with poverty directly, though ironically health care was provided for paupers within the workhouse system. All of these developments had a bearing on the health of the nation whatever the prime motivation for their introduction. More significantly they marked the acceptance of a role for the state in influencing key factors related indirectly and directly to the public health.

This period of early development offered a number of lessons for the future. The British public health movement did reveal the combination of factors needed to promote action. Evidence about the state of health was one element and was provided by the gathering of population statistics and through medical advocacy about the impact of disease and its causes. This was greatly reinforced by the very visible impact of epidemic diseases in a society where individual protection and prevention were not available. The introduction of reforms across a broad front illustrated that even with narrow and modest definitions of health, wider state action could have beneficial effects. Taken together the period illustrates the interrelated factors influencing health and the complex combination of services needed to combat disease.

Two other characteristics of the reforms reflect the circumstances of the time, and have continued to influence the delivery of public services. One was that the system of public provision was new and each new service as it was introduced became the responsibility of a new and separate department of central government, and a new agency of government at the local level where the service was delivered. Eventually local government did develop to take over some functions from the early, independent agencies, but the separation of different services continued in the departmentalized structures adopted by local authorities. The outcome was a pattern of responsibility both in central government and in local government which separated services and those providing them, despite the obvious interrelationship which had brought them into existence.

The other characteristic was the division, and sometimes conflict, between levels of government responsible for different aspects of service and whose joint efforts were essential for any efficient and equitable delivery of public services. Central government could determine national policies and priorities, but always with an eye to the fact that the services would have to be delivered by local agencies, or by local governments independently elected and with taxing powers of their own. The result was a diversity of practice across Britain and across the range of services, and a tendency for central government to make permissive and minimal policy commitments designed to match the willingness and capacity to implement policy of the less cooperative local governments and agencies. This variation was amplified further when services were implemented in detail with wide variations occurring even within single local authority or agency areas.

Evidence about the health of the nation at the turn of the century confirmed the limited gains made by the reforms introduced so far. Charles Booth in London (1889–1903) and Seebohm Rowntree in York (1901), showed the continuing poverty, poor housing, general morbidity and early death in many sectors of the population in two very distinct urban settings, while the Inter-Departmental Committee on Physical Deterioration (1904) confirmed that picture nationally. The gains from public health reforms had been important, but even combined with other developments were not sufficient to combat the impact of continuing social and economic deprivation and inequality. This was reinforced by the fact that more direct aspects of health care, in particular community-based primary care for individuals, were as yet only in their very early years of development. General practice was very limited in its scope and district nursing and health visiting had emerged in the 1860s but were only just beginning the long process of development into their modern form.

DEVELOPMENT IN THE TWENTIETH CENTURY

Early extensions

The impact of this evidence helped to promote a further round of legislation and policy development introduced between 1902 and 1919 widening and deepening the involvement of government in social welfare, health and other services (Hay 1975). Outside health care, education broadened to involve developments in secondary schooling and deepened with further extension of compulsory attendance. Poverty was acknowledged as a cause of many other problems and two of its causes were addressed through the introduction of unemployment insurance and old age pensions. Housing, for so long the object of government inspection to secure standards, took a more central role with the decision to provide council housing after 1919. Government also extended its role into new areas with the provision of school meals for children and the introduction of school medical inspection, forms of primary care which were seen as important preventive measures in relation to disease. Within health care itself, the beginnings of a public system of individual care were made with National Health Insurance in 1911, broadening access to general practitioners through the doctors' 'panel system', though with severe limits being placed on who enjoyed access to this primary care (Gilbert 1966). Health visiting too enjoyed some development with the notification of births and the extension of local authority responsibilities for the service after 1918.

Such incremental movements characterized the development of social policy. They represented real gains in service but their extent was limited by a government unwilling or unable to take more radical steps. That unwillingness arose from the novelty of such provision, the cost of more radical intervention and the conflicts aroused when legislators sought to intervene more directly with those medical, insurance and other interests responsible for providing health care and other services. The First World War delayed further reform and then the economic crises of the 1920s and 1930s reinforced concern about the cost of further development, producing actual reductions in government spending and a delay in further development which might otherwise have been expected to occur.

The Second World War delayed reform still further although it did produce dramatic evidence about the inadequacies of the systems which had been established, about the variability and overall quality of the services provided and the need for reform reflected in evidence about British health. There was evidence of improvement on some fronts, but the revelations produced by mass wartime evacuation from the cities, and medical evidence produced by compulsory conscription into the armed forces, revealed that past policy and action had failed to reach large sections of society, especially the most needy (Titmuss 1950). There was also extensive debate about the character of further reform and a developing consensus for political action to be taken after the war. The case was clear for a further bout of reform and the opportunity to take action came after 1945.

Universal systems

In terms of social welfare the 1940s produced the most extensive and intensive changes in government policy so far. All the public services were overhauled in light of pre-war experience, driven by the general commitment to action prompted by the election of the first majority Labour government. The basis of reform was the Beveridge principle that an integrated attack on the five giants of Idleness, Squalor, Want, Ignorance and Disease should be mounted, acknowledging the historical evidence gained from state involvement in dealing with all five (Beveridge 1942). Idleness would be tackled through economic intervention, Squalor through town planning and a concerted programme of housing renewal, Ignorance through extended universal education and provision for post-compulsory education, Want through universal National Insurance and where this failed a safety net of National Assistance. Each of these was relevant to the wider definition of health, but would also, if successful, impact on the causes of ill-health more narrowly defined and so reduce the incidence of disease. The fifth giant, Disease, would then be tackled directly by the creation of a universal National Health Service. The lessons of history had been learned in respect of the justification for concerted government action on a wide front. They had not yet been learned with regard to how that should be achieved. Nor had they been learned in respect of the scale and quality of provision needed to tackle the legacy of long-term neglect, reinforced by six years of emergency and enforced austerity, or, if they had, the constraints of post-war economic difficulties inhibited what could be done. Implementation lagged behind intention.

One explanation is that the reforms of this period were deeply rooted in the history of welfare provision up to this time. They offered an increment to what had gone before, extended the role of the state in social welfare much more widely, but perpetuated many of the problems that had marked the previous arrangements. One positive extension was the move towards universal provision in most services, with equality of access to services clearly a key goal. In relation to the historical evidence about continuing disparities in relation to all services, but especially in health, despite the presence of developing public services, equal access was an essential condition. Universality was to be sought in a variety of ways, but particularly in health care, it was given important symbolic and practical significance by the decision to provide universal access to primary care, and through primary care to secondary care, and to make health care free of charge at the point of delivery by funding provision from general tax revenue. In principle at least, access for all users would be open and poverty would no longer be the barrier to effective demand for health care which it had once been.

Reforms were less simple on the supply side of health care. Universal free access was associated in health care with the retention of other historical legacies that were less helpful when seeking goals of equality. Despite evidence that many people needed care from a range of public services, the desirability of organizing them in an integrated way that would allow the relations between them to be worked out sensibly and sensitively was not met. Education, housing, social services, and some community health services were provided by local government, though within local government each continued to operate as a separate service reducing the integration inherent in the underlying principles of the programme of reform. Central government continued to be involved in policy development, resourcing and the broad control of each service, though this role continued to be exercised through separate departments of state. Conflicts between central and local governments were not unusual, emerging in education as selection for secondary school became an issue, and recurrently in housing where national interests and those of localities were sometimes in conflict. Social services remained something of a Cinderella service, marginal to the main political debates, with child care dominant and the needs of the elderly and mentally ill much more neglected. On the ground the roles of various professional groups remained confused.

Within health care the position was just as complicated (Watkin 1978). Calls to organize hospitals under local authority control had been rejected and they became the responsibility of regional and local Hospital Boards appointed by central government (with local authority representation). Primary care services within health were organized separately, but were themselves complicated. General practice was separated from hospitals, and GPs enjoyed continuation of the principles established in 1911 having the status of independent contracted practitioners whose contracts with the NHS were organized through local executive councils. Community health services were provided by local authorities, but were marginal to their dominant concerns both financially and politically. They were organized under the aegis of the Medical Officer of Health, reflecting their nineteenth-century beginnings alongside the public health movement.

This structure was made more difficult to operate by the presence of two or three levels of government being involved in the case of local authority services, and several levels of quasi-political control and associated management in the case of health services. These political and managerial complexities were in turn compounded by the fact that some of the fragmentation was the result of powerful pressure from the key professionals in primary care (the GPs), who had been allowed a powerful voice in shaping the organization of the primary care health service which was established. The professional voice in local government, certainly in relation to community health services, was not yet so developed or so articulate, though processes were already beginning in childcare and community nursing after 1946, which would help to create stronger professional voices and a similar fragmented situation within these extended primary care services.

The consequent difficulty of integration was compounded by the failure to deliver adequate resources to meet the demand, let alone the need, already manifest in relation to all these services. Organizational change, extended responsibilities, and a large, known pool of hitherto unmet need, together suggested heavy demands on available resources. Even success on a large scale in relation to Beveridge's other Giants would not have altered that situation, given the goal of equity and the revolution of rising expectations encouraged by reform. This was particularly so where services were universal, free of charge, and where access was seen as a right of citizenship. Need and demand were both encouraged to make themselves known. The resource implications were made more difficult by the problems involved in distribution and redistribution when all services are short of resources and where related services are divided institutionally and their budgets allocated in different ways. In turn this was compounded by the powerful role played by professional staff in taking spending decisions about health care, the division of spending from taxing, and the sharing of taxing powers among different authorities in the case of local government services.

Together these aspects of the reforms meant that national and local governments were often chasing different goals, agencies pursuing different priorities, and provision constantly falling short of expressed demand and visible need. The inevitable consequence was rationing of service, either by systematic means in terms of service entitlement or access, or coincidentally through the everyday operation of services, both of which were in sharp contrast to the hopes expressed in 1946. Waiting lists became the operational device in relation to housing and health care, while in education diversity of quality was evident in schools and selection rationed the places in the more desired grammar schools. All these modes of rationing raise problems but some are more transparent than others. In health care they are usually more opaque, being the product of individual care decisions taken by professional staff and not easily influenced by potential service recipients. Where the latter do have some voice in the decision that voice is known to differ widely in its volume and effect depending on the circumstances of those involved (Hirschman 1970). The evidence about the weaker voices of the sick, the undereducated and the poorly housed is now well established. The inverse relationship between the need for service and the capacity to express demand within the public sector is one key aspect of the failure to achieve equality.

Adapting the structure

Since that momentous period of reform there has been a continuation of the cyclical process of development. Piecemeal changes in different services have continued throughout subsequent years with one short discernible period of more general 'major reform' across the whole range of health and social services. The piecemeal changes addressed particular issues and brought limited improvements to services but inevitably failed to create services that could meet the wider challenge of equitable access, and the more elusive goal of optimizing the outcome of care. Overall standards continued to rise, but evidence of poor levels of health, and inequalities in health care provision continued to emerge, suggesting a need for further reform.

The period of 'major reform', from 1968 until 1974, involved governments of both parties and changes in almost all areas of government activity. These changes reflected a recognition of the structural failings inherited from the nineteenth century and the failure to deal with them successfully in the reforms after 1945. Central government departments were overhauled and several brought together to form large overarching departments responsible for coherent sets of related activities. The potential for integration in this unified political and managerial set up was great. Local government was reformed to reflect the social and economic realities of urban Britain and to create what was essentially a single tier of government for most of the relevant social and health services provided in that sector. The NHS was reorganized to simplify the structure, unify control over some related health services and to create coterminous boundaries between area health authorities (AHA) and local authorities (in almost all cases) in order to ease cooperation between them. Community health services were brought within the AHA but general practice continued as a separate independent sector, inhibiting one of the linkages essential to integration. These changes also reflected a new emphasis on improved efficiency in service delivery which was expected to free up resources for redistribution and to inhibit the tension between levels of government in relation to levels of taxation and of grant, resource allocation and its ultimate use.

Another aspect of the changes addressed the situation in the relevant professions, most visibly in relation to personal social services and child care, but also in community nursing. The evolution of generic social work following the Seebohm Report (Seebohm Committee on Local Authority and Allied Social Services 1968) and of a community orientation in its application, marked a clear change from the previous model of specialization and fragmented practice. This had significant indirect relevance for primary care. More directly, changes in the rules for district nursing opened the way for new working patterns and the development of new roles. In terms of general practice, evidence of low morale and inadequate recruitment was acknowledged with the publication of a GP's Charter in 1965 addressing many of the perceived problems of primary care practice itself (British Medical Association 1965). The Charter dealt with issues of doctor income, investment in premises and arrangements to meet other practice costs but also formalized aspects of the system of GP training. Evidence suggests that it had a distinct impact on many practices, restored morale and paved the way for later developments (Hart 1988). At the same time it reinforced the separation of general practice from the rest of primary care and represented a quite different reform process from that which prevailed in those other areas.

These reforms had been mainly driven by managerial concerns with questions about democratic control and public involvement with the services remaining somewhat marginal. Larger local authorities might be more efficient but seemed unlikely to produce greater public participation and the health service authorities continued to be appointed rather than elected, involving indirect local authority representation and weakening local accountability. General practice remained outside both systems. One result was that although Community Health Councils were established within the NHS in 1974 they were something of an afterthought in the reform process and were given a representative, but not elected, structure, limited resources and a limited role in representing the consumers of health services (Klein and Lewis 1976). Their role in preventing negative decisions about some services was much more significant than any more positive role in the development of policy in relation to health care, and the emphasis on hospitals in the early years was quite pronounced. Judgement about the need for democracy, and about the effectiveness of the existing democratic process, would vary. The rhetoric of the then Conservative government was that managerial efficiency was the key to future development but some argued that it should not be gained at cost to the wider popular involvement essential both in terms of proper account-ability and to legitimize policy development. Others think that formal systems of representation might matter a great deal less if services were better organized to deliver improved quality and more equitable distribution. Certainly the historical evidence from local and central government does not suggest a straightforward relationship between the presence of democratic processes and service quality and equity.

In fact these changes did improve services, but deficiencies remained both in terms of their quality and their distribution. This was acknowledged in a number of ways. Most general was the recognition that the inner cities were a focus of many of the most acute problems of effective service delivery, poorly articulated demand and severe unmet need. The newly restructured system failed to deal with this problem through its normal processes and the result was a series of 'special programmes' aimed at particular services or at more holistic approaches to these inner city areas. Some of these were established with a view to bending main pro-grammes of government spending, but in general normal patterns of service and spend simply co-existed with special programmes. The perceived pressure of demand for speedy and visible political action clearly drove the introduction of special programmes, rather than taking the alternative approach of delaying action while more fundamental assessment of the new structures and their perform-ance took place. In any event, overt acknowledgement that major reorganization might be needed so soon after the debate and upheaval of the early 1970s would have been politically embar-rassing to say the least.

Health authorities had only limited involvement in special pro-grammes, hospitals were seldom exclusively involved in inner cities, and primary care, where inner city services are a problem, was not easily amenable to involvement because of its organization. In the main the NHS as a whole struggled with efforts to adapt within its new structure. Much concern was focused on reforming the well established patterns of resource and service maldistribution, geo-graphically and between medical specialties and sectors of health care. The Resource Allocation Working Party reporting in 1976 proposed major changes in the system for distributing resources within the NHS. Successive efforts were also made to change priorities between secondary and primary care, and between areas of work within these sectors, favouring the elderly and the mentally ill. Much remained as before, however, and the inadequacy of the earlier reforms, and subsequent adaptations, was recognized in the appointment in 1979 of a Royal Commission to investigate the NHS despite general reform only having occurred as recently as 1974.

CONCLUSIONS

This chapter has been concerned with the early phases of the development of the British system of welfare services in general and health services in particular in order to establish the background against which today's reforms with their emphasis on primary care need to be seen and judged. It is clear that phases of reform have successively failed to deliver the holy grail of optimal and equitable health and health care. It is also clear that those phases of reform often involved accurate diagnosis of the conditions that had to be cured and the treatment that would be necessary to achieve improvement. It is equally clear that the political capacity to effect such treatment has been lacking. This reflects the relationships of power and influence within the welfare system. The political parties bring different views to the discussion, and differences between central and local governments make reform difficult. In highly professionalized services, the strength of some of the established professions enables them to resist some fundamental changes, while less developed professions are often weak advocates for changes that might be needed. These factors are reinforced by the sharp divisions between the sectors of care which are relevant to the wider concept of primary care and the problems of integration given their different frameworks of organization, their different resourcing and their varied levels of professionalization.

These themes will be taken up in later chapters but before doing that it is necessary to review the significant next stage of reform. This is particularly important as it reflects a departure from the traditional reform process and a more overt recognition of some of the barriers to change. It also marks a new climate in relation to government attitudes towards the welfare state and its own role in its operation and financing. Together these factors have produced a new model of provision for the NHS and for primary care.

2

A NEW DEPARTURE IN THE 1980s: FORGING NEW LINKS

The Royal Commission on the NHS which reported in 1979 marked something of a watershed in this history of development, though not because its report outlined the changes which drove the subsequent reforms (Merrison 1979). The commission was unusual in being set up so soon after a major restructuring of the NHS, but in other respects operated in quite traditional ways. It maintained the practice of earlier periods, consulting the varied interests involved in health care provision and sustaining the principle from previous reforms of seeking to find a basis for consensual recommendations about change. The result was recommendations for modest structural change, though within the text of the report there was support for more radical principles, but essentially no departure from the prevailing ethos and character of the existing system – this despite evidence of the limited impact of the 1974 changes and the cumulative effect of financial problems since the International Monetary Fund intervention in British public spending plans in the mid-70s.

Evidence that this was a watershed was quickly apparent, not in implementation of the report's recommendations, but in the speed with which a new reform process got under way after 1980 despite a Royal Commission having reported so recently. Financial stringency in the public sector was one major factor but this was not new. What was new was that after 1979 the problem was handled by a government which took a more restricted view of the state's role in welfare compared with that which underlay earlier reforms under both political parties. The years of incremental growth and shared political acceptance of a substantial role for the state in social welfare gave way to an economic philosophy that questioned the appropriateness of high levels of public spending and a political philosophy that favoured a much reduced role for the state.

The process of reform to implement these changes in philosophy has been systematic, and, although it has remained incremental, has had disproportionate impact by being extended over 18 years of single party government. Despite its political philosophy, the Conservative government adopted a very directive role in policy making. The old days of periodic Royal Commissions to examine major changes have gone. So too has the continuing extensive consultation with involved interests, especially of service providers, about possible changes in public policy. These have given way to more limited discussion, mainly within the closed circles of departments of state, sometimes informed by selected contributions from think-tanks or from experts often drawn from outside the public sector. One result has been to accelerate the introduction of new policies. Another has been that government has not proceeded with the traditional large-scale, single reform, but has introduced a series of changes whose cumulative effect over time is fundamentally altering the shape and character of the NHS.

One corollary of this approach to policy making is the difficulty of converting centrally directed changes into reformed practice at the local level, a problem which we have seen beset the previous system despite its very different character. The professional and political interests who would have been consulted in earlier periods are marginalized from the new approach to policy making, but of course remain influential in the implementation of policy. Absence of consultation over policy may lead to weak compliance or even non-compliance, when it comes to implementation. This is more likely in the complex and large-scale public services which are being reformed, especially in health where the legacy is one of fragmentation and where the history of both policy making and implementation have involved high levels of professional input. Most health and social services involve detailed work with individuals, and variation in local practice has been commonplace, in some cases desirable, and largely tolerated, so that the consequent scope for divergence between formal policy and implementation is great. In services such as health, professional judgement and decision lie at the core of both diagnosis and treatment, and are inevitably difficult to control.

Many of the reforms have recognized that fact and have been directed towards giving central government closer direct, or more often indirect, influence over the delivery of services. Structures have been rearranged, intergovernmental relations altered, public spending curbed and directed, and the role, autonomy and power of the professions within the state system directly challenged. With hindsight these interrelated reforms constitute a coherent and radical change in the welfare state though their precise impact on direct services remains to be seen.

A central plank in the approach has been for government to limit the level, and control the direction, of devolved budgets. The apparent threat of resource limitations to service levels and standards has been met by a government campaign aimed at specifying national priority targets and performance standards of its own and arguing that savings can be made by removing the wasteful inefficiencies in existing services. Their analysis argues that expenditure can be cut, but service standards can be maintained, if efficiency is improved, restrictive working practices are removed and work targeted more precisely. In local government this has involved reduced central funding and clear limitations being placed on the level of local taxation. Standard assessments of appropriate levels of service spending have been taken centrally, and local authorities have been required to contract out some aspects of local services to the private sector with competitive tendering. In education this has been associated with increasing budgetary autonomy for individual schools within local education authorities, though significantly accompanied by a centrally directed national curriculum and a requirement for regular testing of pupils. Social service departments have been established as commissioners of services from others as well as continuing as direct providers of some services themselves. In housing, council house-building has effectively stopped, council tenants have been subsidized to become owner-occupiers, and new forms of management have been brought in to council estates. The scope for integrated and coherent planning locally across these services, which we have seen was of great value in developing improved health standards, is greatly reduced although the case for integration remains as strong as ever.

In the health service the philosophy has been the same but the practice different. The structure of the NHS did not involve direct election locally so political differences were less apparent and central political direction was already in place and so much easier to extend. At the same time the scale of the service meant that control over local practice was difficult and professional decisions and action might, it was supposed, inhibit the pursuit of government policy. The result has been a connected series of reforms which interlock to create a new NHS.

The basic reforms of the Conservative government can be summarized as:

1 acceptance that the 'market' provides the best model for optimal and equitable service distribution but that politically the NHS cannot be privatized. In consequence a 'quasi-market' has been established to manage the supply of, and demand for, local health services;

2 recognition that this market model cannot operate with individuals as purchasers, and so must depend on intermediaries (GPs and health authorities) acting on behalf of the public and requiring competing sources of service provision from which to choose if the market is to function competitively;

3 recognition that professional domination of much policy and decision making must be overcome for the model to work, and that, taken together with the need for efficiency gains in service provision, this would require much higher levels of managerial control over resource use within the new NHS;

4 all of these changes are undertaken in the interests of patients and with a view to enhanced patient choice. In the absence of the conventional individual basis for the market, patients' rights and expectations would need to be safeguarded through the introduction of the *Patient's Charter* – 'quasi-consumerism' in a 'quasi-market';

5 all of these changes should be associated with centrally defined operational targets, performance standards and details of performance published where possible so that government targets can be seen to be met (or missed) and purchasers and providers make enlightened decisions according to good information.

AN NHS MARKET

Central to the new structure is acceptance of the view that the market is the best medium for determining the provision and distribution of goods and services. This contrasts sharply with the historical development of state welfare as a substitute for a market that failed to meet perceived key needs in social welfare. Because of its origins the health service was seen to have placed no sensible limit on what could and should be done and so on what could and should be spent. For the patient/consumer the service was free at the point of delivery in order to secure equitable access. For the professional working in the system decisions in response to demand were not concerned with considerations of cost. The implications of that combination can be seen throughout the history of the NHS and were the subject of ongoing debate. Of course budgets could not support all the treatments which were possible and desirable but the imbalance between effective demand and available resources was met by the use of extensive waiting lists for treatment in secondary care. In primary care it resulted in reduced consultation times, probably led to prescribing as a substitute for more considered case management, and the quality of care would have been higher with less pressure of demand. The system worked well in treating serious acute cases which needed to move through primary into secondary care. It coped much less well with the widespread, chronic health problems which arose in the community and needed to be treated at home. It found the redistribution of resources particularly difficult within and between existing patterns of primary and secondary care and there were problems coping with expressed demand (Resource Allocation Working Party 1976).

These processes have been replaced by an artificial market in which agencies within the health service became purchasers or providers, or in the case of some GPs, both purchaser and provider (Le Grand and Bartlett 1994). The resources for this market to operate are distributed through a conventional national system but the allocation to those providers of secondary care and some community services now depends on formal annual contracts for their services negotiated with purchasers who hold the NHS budgets. Purchasers include the local health authorities (HAs) acting for large localities, and where they have volunteered to do so, general practice fundholders. The latter have budgets which cover the costs of their own services, purchase of some parts of secondary care, and purchasing has been steadily extended to include aspects of community health care and in some cases total fundholding where all services are included. As a corollary of these changes hospitals and community health service providers were established as independent trusts securing 'market competition' on the supply side and allowing purchasers in many areas some discretion about where they place contracts for care.

In essence provision has ceased to be based on a guaranteed annual budget to the provider and has become subject to the variability of a dispersed contractual process with possible shifts of custom from one hospital or community trust to another over time. General practices cease to be able to refer without limit as demand dictates and are constrained in fundholding and more generally by the limitations of their own, or of HA budgets, and by the character and quality of the contracts that have been negotiated. The intention was that resources would follow patient needs and interests and that the spur of potential income or loss of income would stimulate development and good practice among both purchasers and providers. It would also mean that the pattern of care for a patient would lie much more within the control of primary care than had traditionally been the case. Reform stopped short of freeing this system from control however and there is much scope for central intervention if, as has happened, providers run out of money because of contractual factors or purchasers retain 'profit' from their allocated budgets. The market principle has been adopted but has been constrained in its operation.

MANAGERIALISM

One of the more controversial aspects of the changes has been the injection of an emphasis on management into the organization of care. This fits closely with the argument that the service has been inefficient, and undermanaged historically. Good management can raise efficiency levels, but in a labour intensive and professionalized service like health the implications of change are both visible and significant. Management has to be applied at various levels including broad resource allocations, but when it is applied at the point of service delivery where traditionally a great deal of latitude has been enjoyed by professionals then it can create serious tensions. If management is seen by the professions as one element in a strategy aimed at curbing their autonomy, and inevitably involving clinical judgements having to be modified, then of course it will be seen as threatening. If it tries to do this indirectly, through the introduction of performance standards or of new processes for resource allocation, it will ultimately have the same effect. If it does not do this then the efficiency gains and redistribution expected may not occur. In all these cases it can and does lead to sharp conflict between managers and professionals about who should control the service.

The development of management began as early as 1983 with the Griffiths Report (1983) and has been integrated into subsequent structural reforms and into the detailed organization of practice. The management revolution is reflected in the creation of the NHS Management Executive with its much clearer focus on central direction and management of the whole service. This has been reaffirmed in the changes in the regional structure introduced in 1996 and is reflected in the periodic reorganization of the intermediate levels of the service creating and then merging the HAs and the Family Health Service Authorities (FHSAs). These changes have carried down to the local level and are to be found in the increased emphasis on management in the operation of the new trusts. Recruitment to Trust Boards reflects this emphasis, bringing professionals onto them in managerial roles and recruiting non-executive expertise from the business sector to improve management in relation to the new internal market.

An associated feature of this change has been the creation of managerial opportunities for medical staff, within the management structure of the hospital trusts. The creation of clinical directorates has given explicit managerial roles, and responsibilities, to some doctors, marking a major change in orientation from their less formal managerial roles in the past. Management of a clinical team continues but is now undertaken in the context of a wider corporate concern and with a devolved responsibility for finance. This has produced tensions for those appointed as they straddle the boundary where clinical and managerial issues meet and where the compromises inevitable in a resource-limited service have to be faced. The implications of the contractual purchaser/provider process have added greatly to the demands of the task.

These changes do not have such a direct parallel in primary care or general practice. The tradition of a senior GP managing a practice continues in many cases though often with quite a limited view of that managerial role. The potential significance of the changes can be seen in fundholding, however, where the increased managerial demands have led to the appointment of a new and effective type of practice manager. Extension of that model would echo the changes in secondary care, and highlight even more acutely the issues of management in a professional setting. Of course for nursing and social work the concept of management and of being managed, are well established, though the transition from professional to manager in those areas is clearly difficult and confirms the difficulty of adopting this model more widely within the NHS. In addition the role of FHSAs, and now the HAs, has been strengthened with the clear intention that they should play a managerial and supervisory role intended to influence the climate within general practice and directly condition practice itself. The Audit Commission Report on FHSAs clearly outlines this potential, 'extending their role to act as development agencies', needing to act as 'commissioners of services' and to undertake performance review in general practice (Audit Commission 1993). All of these are tasks with significant implications for the operation and conduct of primary care and, if they are carried through, the professional, managerial and service implications could be profound.

FRAGMENTATION

After many years of discussion about the problems of fragmentation within the NHS and between health and other related services, the new system is more fragmented than ever although tempered in its effect by other changes. In the old days of centralized service planning, securing cooperation and compliance in local delivery was the great challenge. Reforms were consistently aimed at removing gaps, resolving boundary difficulties, securing integration and changing priorities. The new system does not accept that traditional model of centralized planning, rightly recognizing that it did not work well, although it does impose targets and priorities determined centrally. In its place it sees market processes as controlling the delivery of services through the interaction of purchaser and provider institutions. For the market to operate those functions have to be separated, and competition among providers and purchasers is necessary for efficiency and improved performance. The result has been the development of an extensive range of localized, partly autonomous agencies, although coupled with a good deal of market regulation through central direction and oversight.

Community care is an area where the reforms have promoted a more integrated approach to care and with it the need for a more managerial approach (Øvretveit 1993). Management may not be new to local government as it is to general practice, but the role of social services in commissioning and planning community care is, and now gives them a managerial input to general practice which was never present in the past. The impact of this change is magnified by the fact that the new system started properly with the aim of providing high quality care packages. These were expensive, and coupled with the revelation of need by the new system, have revealed serious resource limitations that are inhibiting service provision and having wider effects within the NHS. The formal split between health and social care budgets in meeting need has led to conflicts over the apportionment of costs, rather than encouraging an integrated view being taken of cases. The results are producing predictable tensions between carers and managers, but also between primary and secondary care as discharges are held up by the need for community care, and between sectors of what was intended to become a seamless primary care system. The efficiency gains of managed integration of care may be forthcoming where they can be applied. The structure introduced to achieve that efficiency may have the effect of revealing unmet need, creating tensions in the supply of service and leaving waiting lists for care as one very visible legacy. The sequel will need to be a shared engagement with those implications if the result is not to degenerate into a simple loss of service for a large number of clients. The imposed marriage between sectors is no doubt producing exciting examples of innovative shared working, but it is also revealing the difficulties of operating the new system with the present organizational arrangements and more importantly with the present levels of resource.

PATIENTS AS CUSTOMERS

In a conventional market for health care the patient would be the customer and pay directly for the service as is the case with private medicine. The NHS reforms have not adopted that market model as has been seen. This is mainly because the political implication might be drawn that the NHS was ceasing to exist as a public service and was being privatized, or potentially being made accessible to privatization, and in any event the public funding of a conventional market for health would be extremely complex. Instead HAs and fundholding general practices act as surrogate consumers on behalf of their populations or their registered patients. The need for good information in the quasi-market has led the Conservative government to establish performance criteria about practice and to publish details of aspects of the performance of hospital trusts. The resulting league tables provide some evidence in the market place and purchasers are expected to monitor performance around their own contractual experience. This is intended to influence decisions about where purchasers place their contracts for service and about changes in those contracts as time goes by. The use of performance criteria of this kind, particularly in a transparent and widely publicized way, creates a framework for wider judgements about health care and is another form of implicit intervention in areas which were traditionally seen as autonomous professional activity.

At the same time, the new system and the rhetoric that surrounds the operation of the quasi-market, despite their indirect operation, do have some direct implications for those who use the services. This is reflected in the widespread development of the concept of the Citizen's Charter, and a specific *Patient's Charter* for the NHS (Department of Health 1995b). In essence the charter offers citizens a series of standards of service that they should expect from their health services and avenues through which they may complain should those standards not be met. These standards relate mainly to the non-clinical, administrative aspects of the service and are outlined as national performance criteria by central government. They are no less significant for that, including issues such as waiting times for consultation and for treatment, but they exclude issues associated with the character and quality of the care being delivered. While they leave professional judgement out of the account, the existence of the charter, and the requirement to publish it widely, may encourage patients to take a more demanding line about non-charter issues as well. The expectation is that consumer pressure through this mechanism will add to other pressures in the market to ensure that providers comply with consumer wishes. One limitation of this kind of approach is that it facilitates patients' complaints about inadequacies in service, but only after the event, leaving unanswered many questions about the consumer voice in relation to service development and priorities.

PRIMARY CARE

At the heart of the Conservative government's reforms in the NHS has been the clear intention to break with the historical traditions outlined in Chapter 1 and in so doing to create a primary care-led NHS. The history of the NHS confirms the logic of seeking such a central role for primary care and may even be seen as little more than the formalization of the previous *de facto* position. The ambiguous response to the policy, certainly within general practice, suggests that achievement of the necessary changes involved may not be so easy. The ambiguity reflects widespread anxiety among GPs about the implications of change in primary care and uncertainty about what playing a leading role in the NHS might mean. For some their reaction involves little more than a wish that nothing

should change. For many more it reflects a wish to retain the traditional model of primary care that is seen as inconsistent with the
reforms which 'many of us believe deeply . . . have been at best mis-
guided, and at worst malevolent' (Heath 1995: 52). For others, there
is acceptance both of the need for change and for some or all of the
particular changes that have been introduced. Some acknowledge
that primary care needs to change, in terms of the services that it
offers, the way in which it is organized and the range of people who
will be involved in its delivery and management. A few have gone
further, adopted the changes, and begun to adapt their practices to
take advantage of the opportunities which they see arising.

This broad mixture of opposition, uncertainty, acceptance and
keen adoption is not untypical of the traditional response to change
within the NHS (Stocking 1985). It partly reflects the success of
general practice in resisting change in the past and is therefore a
reaction to the perceived lack of consultation with the profession
in the development of the reforms. It also reflects anxiety about
what is involved and about how best some of the aims might be
achieved. This has been clearly evident in the rhetoric about
reform, and in the reaction to a number of detailed changes in
policy ranging across an extended primary care. These policies have
addressed three separate issues. One has been the relationship
between the different agencies involved in an extended version of
primary care. Another has been the relationship and the balance of
work between secondary care in the hospitals and primary care in
the community. A third has involved direct changes in primary care,
narrowly defined in this case as traditional general practice.

Community care, introduced in 1991, takes a long-standing
policy of closing the large Victorian mental hospitals and moving
patients into the community and extends it into a more general
policy of care for psychiatric patients and the elderly. In doing so
it has imposed links between separate agencies to develop systematic pre-planning of community care involving formal arrangements for multidisciplinary working with complex budgetary
implications between social service departments and general practice. In some cases this has worked well, but in others, far from creating an integrated model of care in the community, it has led to
mutual acrimony about whether the care being provided is 'social'
or 'health' and consequently which budget should fund the necessary action. Inadequate and divided resourcing has limited the
benefit of a major policy to extend the concept of integrated
primary care.

Reform of health care in London illustrates another strand in primary-led development. Following the report of the Tomlinson Committee (1992) the government took a bold decision to reduce the number of hospital beds in London, in the process closing, or merging a number of famous hospitals. Developments in conventional primary care were intended to compensate for the loss, providing alternative care in the community in much more economical ways. This clear shift in the balance of provision between primary and secondary care is central to the concept of a primary-led NHS, but the response in London has been a traditional rearguard defence by the hospitals, a failure to provide the necessary resources for primary care, and a consequent fear that primary care will not be able to meet the new demands.

Less visible than these formal changes but driven by budgetary pressures in the new quasi-market has been the dramatic change in the character of hospital care. The sharp increase in day-case treatment in hospitals may be seen within the new trusts as marking a significant increase in their efficiency and contributing towards meeting the prime political target of reducing patient waiting lists. The corollary has been a move of the continuing care for such patients into the community after early discharge, placing heavy burdens on primary care services without always providing new resources to meet them.

Within primary care itself a number of major changes have been introduced. In some ways the most significant was the introduction in 1990 of a new contract for GPs working within the NHS. This was significant partly for what it required general practice to do, and partly because it created, for the first time, a situation in which it was possible for government to influence directly what GPs did in their practices. The contract placed increased emphasis on health promotion and disease prevention, broadening the traditional focus of general practice. More importantly it introduced payments to stimulate such development, relating them directly to the government health targets outlined in *The Health of the Nation* (Secretary of State for Health 1992). Clearly such targeting is a crude way to address complex issues as is illustrated in occasional cases of GPs tampering with patient lists in order to achieve targets. It also sought to stimulate the employment of additional staff, and promoted the establishment of a range of clinics to pursue the policy of health promotion. Evidence suggests that these aims were achieved although the longer term implications remain to be seen (Hannay *et al.* 1992).

Much more controversial in terms of public debate has been the introduction of fundholding into general practice since 1991. This was a voluntary scheme that provided those GPs who volunteered to take part with a budget to pay for the drugs they prescribe, the staff they employ, and 20 per cent of the health care their patients receive from hospitals and community services. From small beginnings the scheme has extended to involve almost one quarter of all general practices serving more than half of all patients. It has also been extended on a pilot basis to allow some practices, or consortia, to purchase all the care that their patients need. At the same time there have been developments introducing methods for involving GPs in the HA purchasing of services, avoiding the implications of fundholding, which some of them oppose.

As with all reforms, and especially those introduced on a voluntary basis and into a system changing in many other ways, the evidence about its impact is not yet as clear as it might be. However, the system has been monitored and the evidence to date suggests that there are good practices who

> have thought carefully about what they can achieve by becoming fundholders, are well managed and achieve a lot for their patients ... but such practices are rare, and a more important question concerns the others. The majority of fundholding practices do not appear to be especially good at management and networking or achieving a large number of benefits for patients.
>
> (Audit Commission 1996b: 106)

There is evidence here of the historical model for the introduction of change being applied. The voluntary principle may be necessary in an area where there is considerable division of opinion, but in leaving implementation to those already within the system, the impact of reform may be weakened and the pace of reform slowed considerably. If the quasi-market is to work then it needs the surrogate purchasers to operate effectively if some patients are not to be disadvantaged. The evidence of varied practice characterized the old system, but the reform was designed to promote improvement, not change the distribution and causes of inequality.

A key change associated with both the contract and with fundholding has been change in the pattern of staffing within primary care, and particularly in the teams working within general practices. Their effect has been to increase the employment of practice nurses, and of other professional staff, working within or attached to general practice. This in turn has raised questions about patterns of work, allocation of responsibility and management of resources, which were once relatively simple but are becoming quite complex. Not everyone is dealing with them effectively. Current evidence about stress among GPs and related difficulties in retaining some doctors and recruiting others indicates how difficult adaptation is proving.

CONCLUSIONS

These associated reforms, brought in over a relatively short period of time, provide a new model NHS. Starfield's (1992) goals have not been rejected, indeed they continue to figure in the rhetoric of debate, but a new system has been established for their achievement. Not only is it new, it is also largely untested, and successful implementation will pose a considerable challenge to those working within the system. Given the history of health care, and in particular of primary care, and the continuing demands and constraints on the services, a closer look is needed at the implications of the new system for those working within it. This must start from a clearer understanding of primary care and a fuller analysis of its provision than has been used in the past if the structures, processes, roles and procedures are to adapt successfully to the new NHS.

3

PRIMARY CARE TODAY

The argument advanced here is that the Conservative government's reforms in the NHS reflect recognition of some of the lessons of the history outlined in Chapter 1, but appear to have ignored significant others, or intend to address them in indirect ways. They were right in recognizing that the existing system was limited in its capacity to deliver significant change, and that key reforms would have to address greater integration and have to challenge traditional patterns of professional dominance of decision making. The designers of the reforms were also right about the centrality of primary care in the NHS. It is not yet clear that they were right about the appropriateness of the market model in achieving those ends, or in the capacity of a new managerial cadre to deliver change on the scale required. They were wrong in supposing that a new model of practice could be introduced without greater reference to the factors which would condition its implementation. The reforms have tackled the obvious shortcomings of the existing structure by seeking to stimulate change through the external dynamic of the market process, but in doing so have failed to address structural and cultural issues which may need to change if reform is to work.

This may reflect an understandable wish not to become involved in the sorts of battles inherent in tackling those issues, or from a more cynical standpoint it could be a case where the fundamental outcome is less significant than the symbolic significance of appearing to tackle a range of related issues. More Machiavellian still would be an interpretation which saw reform, assuming a failure to deliver on goals of equality and optimization, as paving the way for a more radical change consistent with the new mechanisms but involving more fundamental changes in the NHS. Whether any of these objectives apply, or some other overall objective, history suggests that the failures of the past were less about intention and more about implementation so that we should be suspicious of reforms which claim such high capacity to change patterns of behaviour.

It must be recognized in saying this that the goals of optimal health and equitable care that Starfield (1992) outlined may not be as widely shared as she supposed. If the outcome desired is more narrow, or more limited, then the reforms may well be adequate. If economy in terms of health service costs is the key objective then optimal health care and equitable distribution are unlikely to be successfully achieved. If the goal is to curb professional power then the quality of patient care may be put at risk. If the aim is to transfer clear accountability and responsibility for delivery of care from those who fund onto those who deliver, that is from politicians to managers and professionals, then increased fragmentation may be a necessary price. But if the goal really is optimal and equitable health care then the past does offer guidance about other reforms that might reinforce those now in place in securing success.

Before examining that issue it is necessary to achieve some clarity about what is meant when we talk of primary care, a clarity that is lacking in much of the debate around reform. This applies both to the ideas and concepts that underlie primary care and to the current pattern of primary care provision, both of which must condition any successful effort at reform.

Despite the current vogue for a political rhetoric that places primary care at the centre of a reformed NHS the evidence about it is remarkably sparse. At the practical level this reflects the history of fragmentation and division within health and related care, which greatly complicate the material evidence about what is being provided and by whom. This is reinforced by the dominance in general practice of an individualistic ethic which at its most extreme comes close to defining every case by its uniqueness and widely divergent practice as legitimate, both of which limit the availability of evidence on which to base coherent judgement. It also reflects the professional commitment to confidentiality which on the one hand may protect patients, but can also inhibit the gathering of key data about the public's health and about professional performance, as well as inhibiting patient influence. As John Fry (1993: v) observed

It is truly amazing that Europe's largest employer, the NHS, with over one million workers, and with an annual cost of over £30 billion, should have existed and survived with so little available and published information and so few data for analysis, audit and action.

He then went on to seek out what information was available in order to clarify the pattern of existing care, an essential requirement for making a legitimate contribution to the debate.

THE CHARACTER OF PRIMARY CARE

Before doing that we need first to consider what is meant by primary care. Definitions range widely in their scope from those concerned narrowly with the delivery of medical care to those that adopt a wider and more inclusive concern with health maintenance and consequently embrace much more than the purely medical. This issue of scope is strongly related to the institutional developments of earlier periods and definitions often reflect the character of the formal context in which the debate is being held. The broad arena of health care policy debate excludes a wide range of services that are relevant to health, and in the particular case of social welfare, some that perhaps share many characteristics with core primary care. The narrow arena of primary care was historically concerned exclusively with general practice, and that concern came to define the debate, and allowed it to be conducted within the profession on terms that they determined. Primary care was what general practitioners provided. The difficulty was that what they did varied widely and there was clear difficulty in agreeing what the core activity was and even more difficulty about how it might be assessed.

The debate now has moved on from that position with much discussion about the primary care team, with the Royal College of General Practitioners (RCGP) accepting this wider scope of definition. Interestingly this wider notion of primary care does not readily spread over into debate about the organization and management of care, but sees the team as attached to the GP who in turn is the key determinant of what team members will do. GPs have not in the main considered radical alternative forms of organization, so discussion of teams has often operated within the limits set by the accepted model of general practice.

In order to avoid that institutional trap it is important to consider ways in which the scope of primary care might be determined by its essential character rather than by its institutional setting. We are helped in this by Starfield's excellent discussion of primary care, albeit that she is working from a traditional medical perspective. Analysing a wide range of earlier work she establishes four key elements; accessibility, continuity, comprehensiveness and coordination which she argues distinguish primary care (Starfield 1992). In her discussion she is concerned with the distinction between primary medical care and secondary or tertiary care within the health services. In our discussion the concern is to examine these characteristics more widely in relation to the other services, both medical and social, which find a place in many primary health care teams.

In the context of the NHS accessibility looks straightforward. Everyone registers with a GP and enjoys the right of direct access to that GP when in need of care. There is no charge at the point of contact with the GP so a key historical limitation on access is thereby removed. The geography of provision is highly dispersed with an average list of patients for a GP numbering only 1900, ensuring ease of access to consult in all except perhaps the most remote rural areas. Accessibility is confirmed in the pattern of use of the service with a very high volume of consultation taking place. There are people who do not use the service, or use it less readily, but that is more likely to reflect their self-perceived need rather than the inaccessibility of care.

Interesting in relation to this formal model of access are a number of trends in patient behaviour and in the provision of general practice. In terms of patients there has been a recent marked increase in the tendency to self-refer directly to accident and emergency (A and E) departments in hospitals rather than proceed through the accessible intermediacy of the GP. The reasons for this are a matter of current research interest, but may be related to changes in the availability of some GPs and particularly of a known GP. The pattern of surgery hours and the unavailability of a preferred GP may limit patients' perception of ease of access and make a visit to A and E every bit as acceptable as a visit to an 'unknown' doctor even in one's own registered practice. This is amplified outside normal surgery hours where the establishment of alternatives to 24-hour care by one's own doctor has changed the concept of access quite substantially. Indeed that concept was already outmoded by the advent of large group practices, the sharing of on-call duties between practices and the extensive use of deputizing services.

At the same time other changes in general practice raise questions about the principle of accessibility. The appointment of practice nurses, and changes in the character of contact with practices (clinics and checks rather than consultations) is changing the pattern of who is seen by the patient and the character of the service received when they visit. Experiments with triage systems in the new extended primary care team set-up are sometimes placing nurses in a gatekeeping role *vis-á-vis* the team, placing the doctor behind the gate rather than in the role of first-access gate-keeper. At the same time, receptionists continue to play a role as gatekeepers over access into primary care, sometimes exercising their own judgement and experience to protect medical staff or applying protocols designed by the GPs within their practice to govern access. More fundamentally, the ending of out-of-hours care and the creation of large cooperatives to provide deputizing services has attenuated the concept of access, making it a rather different criterion from its original conception.

Once one moves to this kind of situation then the GP in principle becomes much more like other professionals offering services in the community, although traditional popular perceptions of, and the stigma associated with some of those other services, limit the direct demand placed on them. District nurses operate on referral, but do provide easy access for patients, with domiciliary visiting moving the issue of access to a quite different plane. The same is true of health visitors where the legal requirements of some aspects of the role remove the need for referral and go well beyond the realms of patient determined voluntary access that apply in general practice. The distinction between their work with children and with the elderly is clear evidence of this factor and of the attitudes of the elderly towards care and of professionals towards the elderly. Social workers too are not inaccessible though they are usually reached through a referral system with only limited client self-referral to what many regard as a stigmatizing service. That stigma arises in part from the perceptions held about what social workers can do on the part of those who refer clients, and the client experience that results from 'wrong' referrals. Creation of the opportunity for more direct access, and for self-referral, might reveal a quite different pattern of service and create new attitudes towards the service.

If accessibility is a changing criterion, what can be said of conti-nuity? Continuity is conditional in part upon access, but is more sig-nificantly affected by the process involved in contact with primary care over time. Once again formal registration creates an impres-sion of continuity and in many cases this does apply, with patients seeing the same doctor over time and benefiting from the personal knowledge and contextual awareness which that brings. But for many that is not the case. A different doctor is seen on different visits, and the more limited scale of house calls inhibits some of the contextual awareness that has been seen as an important feature of continuity in primary medical care. This causes Starfield to consider the issue of patient records and their role in delivering continuity. It is true that the record is available to all the doctors in the practice, and to the locum, but out of hours this may be difficult and the quality of records and recording becomes highly significant to effective continuity of care. Even when available the record is limited. The quality of note taking, and the consistency across a range of carers become issues of importance. So too do those informal factors which would be known by a doctor providing continuity of care but which may not always find a place in the medical record. This applies even more acutely to any record of social care which a patient may be experiencing, and to aspects of secondary health care which may not be recorded within the primary care record. These potential limitations must cause us to rethink the idea of continuity and suggest that other professions need to be seen as elements in the continuing care being provided, especially where chronic conditions are involved and the likely recurrent need is for only limited medical service. The development of the idea of patient-held records reflects this broad debate and could create a situation in which the patient provides the effective continuity independent of which agency is involved.

With or without effective records the character of care offered by other primary care professions also involves elements of continuity though without the formality of registration it takes on an apparently more limited character. Social workers do take clients through extended episodes of care, apart from residential care, and team working together with formal supervision of field workers can produce continuity even where individual staff change. The same is true for much chronic care, which is delegated to nursing staff and only comes back to the doctor if crises occur. District nursing and health visiting share these characteristics of continuity. Area-based team work extends this idea of continuity in that future episodes of care will be handled by the same department and possibly by the same staff, so that the contrast with most patients of general practice becomes less distinct.

If continuity poses some problems, comprehensiveness is even more difficult. In Starfield's (1992) usage it means that the primary care doctor is able either to provide directly for a patient's needs or has the diagnostic skill and the knowledge of other services to act as an effective gatekeeper to them. In relation to core medical conditions this is not difficult although opinion about the appropriateness and quality of much referral to secondary care is divided. GPs do, however, share a lengthy common training with their specialist colleagues, develop extensive experience of common conditions and continuing treatment of them, making appropriate referrals likely. Where the range of need widens to include less common conditions, or newly emerging areas such as psychiatric care, the issue becomes more complex and the quality of referral less certain. Where the need is for a service outside medicine referral becomes much more difficult. A recent study of GP fundholding found coincidentally that 'many GPs do not even know what their non-medical colleagues are doing or which of their patients were being seen by whom' (Glennerster *et al*. 1994).

This can lead to definitions of primary care, and indeed of patient need, being limited by the awareness and understanding of professionals. Lack of awareness can lead to inappropriate referral, or to no referral at all being made where a gatekeeper is unaware of what might be available within one of the parallel services. More fundamentally this failure to refer, or inappropriate referral, can direct or inhibit the development of those other services as expressed demand reinforces some activity while unexpressed demand limits the information needed to stimulate alternative service development. The development of the range of primary care services in part reflects the historical patterns of usage dictated by the dominant gatekeeping profession. Their referral patterns often dictate the service response, which may not reflect the training and skill of the professions involved in these associated services.

This problem is compounded by the overlaps in terms of their perceived skills and competence among the professions involved. All the professions share elements of concern with aspects of continuing care, and all define the quality of their interaction with patients and clients as the basis of their work. Each has core skills which overlap less, but professional development has often been marked by an extension of that core into areas of work and roles that are shared with others.

Coordination takes this problem onto another level. It implies a role for someone within primary care to bring together a very wide array of information about the patient's current condition and background experience and to decide about any necessary treatment and care in that context. Inevitably this involves high quality recording of information but also high levels of good communication across the comprehensive array of services just discussed. There is much discussion of communication in general practice, but almost always it is about the patient–doctor relationship rather than about the interagency and interprofessional communication that lies at the base of any coordinated service. Coordination goes further, however. It implies a role for the GP, or for someone in the team, in managing the wide pattern of care which may be relevant to a patient. It is not consistent with referral being the endpoint of responsibility. Fundholding, and the contracting process it involves in the new quasi-market, has introduced a greater element of continuity, and implicit coordination, into the relationship between primary and secondary care, and experimentally into a wider range of care provision. Evidence about practice suggests that the care management role inherent in that process varies widely and has not yet permeated the new system, let alone extended into the alternative purchasing systems outside fundholding.

This concept of the GP as coordinator of care reflects the long historical dominance of medicine in the context of professional services providing health and social care. The coordinating role falls to the dominant as it cannot readily be undertaken interprofessionally without the status that medicine has enjoyed. That situation is changing of course as other professions emerge into maturity and is interesting when set against the conduct of the new system of community care. There the social work department carries the formal responsibility for coordination, in theory directing the input of the GP as much as that of social work staff. It is also interesting that in this case the function is carried by managers in social services rather than by professional social workers delivering the care. This issue of role definition will be considered later.

It seems from this review that there is a good conceptual case for extending the scope of primary care to embrace a wide range of professionals working in the community and to those supporting them in their work. This is not merely a matter of attaching other professions to general practice but recognizes the interchangeability of several professions in providing many primary care services.

CRITERIA IN THE MARKET PLACE

Over and above these professional criteria for the definition of primary care are another set of criteria which do not define the practice but that frame its delivery and define its success. These have become prominent in the reforms since the early 1980s to the extent that some would argue that they now dominate to the exclusion of the more substantive service criteria considered above. One criterion, present in the past, but mainly left to the professions, involves the question of service quality, which has become much more a matter of public debate. Related to quality and in some ways qualifying judgement about it are the related criteria of equality, equity, efficiency and effectiveness.

Quality is an elusive issue in the context of primary care. The formal characteristics of the system, and the *Patient's Charter* criteria, are clear about quality in relation to accessibility and eligibility, and for broadly administrative matters, but have little to say about the quality of care provided. The nature of all primary care makes this difficult. Care and treatment are largely a matter of direct contact between patient and professional, with the patient relatively weak in such a relationship, and with confidentiality limiting external professional review of individual practice. Formal supervision may go some way towards independent judgement about practice, but it is missing in the case of GPs and not always very effective in the other professions where it is applied. This makes the character of professional education and training of prime importance in securing standards of practice. The debate about professional accreditation, and about continuing reaccreditation, particularly in general practice, confirms that there is limited agreement about the core of practice, the character of best practice and the desirability (or even possibility) of judging such matters at all. The implications for the patient are obvious.

The absence of reliable evidence about quality makes it more difficult to deal with the four other criteria. It does not invalidate them, but does mean that the operational measures used in applying such criteria are limited to the measurable aspects of practice, which usually means the administrative aspects. Bearing that in mind, equality is widely used as an evaluatory criterion in reference to the NHS. The removal of formal barriers to access to care created a system intended to respond only to health care need, but which in its operation failed to secure equality. Equality of access is itself elusive, and even if it could be delivered, the variations in service then received within the NHS and within primary care would limit its effect. Evidence is now widely available about inequalities in health and about inequalities in health services and about the inverse care law that continues to apply (Hart 1971; Townsend *et al.*

1988). The distribution of GPs and of group practices and more elaborate health centres, together with evidence about nursing and social work provision, confirm the systematic patterns of inequality despite them having been the object of much reform effort.

Equity is a criterion that takes us somewhat further along the evaluatory path. It is defined by the degree to which services are provided according to need and not mediated by other factors which may affect accessibility. Need here is a complex issue with a wide array of factors giving rise to ill-health and as a result determining what action might be taken. This is made more difficult by the question of who determines that a need exists (Bradshaw 1972). The normative views of doctors and other professionals about need have traditionally determined the provision of service, despite evidence of quite divergent opinions being held. The felt needs of patients may be what brings them to consult primary care but those presenting problems are translated by professionals into diagnoses often dictated by the availability of services. It is clear that much definition of normative need is conditioned by perceived resource availability, knowledge of other services and the view taken about the availability of professionals' time. Comparative need is well established in debate among public health specialists, but within primary care the character of provision makes it a difficult concept to invoke when deciding about service.

Effectiveness relates to notions of need and is concerned with the degree to which any service provided deals with a particular need. A wide variety of perspectives may be adopted in looking at effectiveness, conditioned in large measure by the time perspective being adopted. In the short run of course many needs presented in primary care are minor, or of a self-limiting character so that effectiveness is almost guaranteed. Others are more complex. In the acute cases, referral is the effective response with ultimate judgement being reserved for the outcome of the secondary care provided. In chronic cases, continuing care is the proper response but wider issues than the simple provision of primary care treatment are often called into play. Effectiveness might be considered as providing treatment when required and mitigating the limiting effects of a condition. Within primary care this perspective usually involves the attention of a widely defined professional team. On the other hand it could be considered over a longer time period and involve more direct engagement with causal factors, such as housing and education, usually perceived as being outside the direct influence of primary care. Health education, immunization and screening are variants of this but they do lie within the province of primary care and do form part of the evaluation of the service.

Efficiency is the criterion that links effectiveness with the resource inputs involved in providing services. In effect it involves a cost–benefit analysis of primary care with optimal service at least cost being the preferred model. Two problems arise in applying this kind of analysis. One is the wide range of primary care inputs involved in some cases, compounded by the fact that other non-care factors may be influencing the outcome of treatment and care. The other is that the outcome may itself not be clear and certainly not always easy to assess. Given the concept of continuity in primary care there are difficult issues involved in determining when care has ended and so when evaluation should take place. The self-limiting episodes provide a useful illustration of the difficulties involved. On the one hand it may be cheapest and most efficient not to treat in such cases, though there may be side benefits to treatment which ought to be taken into account. In the same way, a decision to treat in such cases, for whatever reason, may build up patient expectations and imply commitment to future action that go well beyond the costs of a particular episode of care. The need for long term considerations to be taken into account even in what are often short term cases is central to primary care with its inbuilt continuity and the important possibility of mutual education between patient and professional.

CURRENT PROVISION

Before turning to examine ways in which more effective reform in primary care might be engaged, it is essential to have a clear understanding of what currently goes on within both the narrow and the more extended idea of primary care. This is made difficult by the absence of good quality data about primary care, and the individuality and confidentiality of provision which militate against easy characterization of practice. It is really a matter of examining available evidence to arrive at some picture of practice and being careful in drawing conclusions. This is particularly the case when one wishes to move beyond consideration of the professionals involved to talk about the system, and importantly about the 'practice' or other unit of provision. Available evidence can give us some idea of the scale of primary care, both on the supply side in terms of professional and other staff, and on the demand side in terms of the use made of the service by the public. The first is perhaps easier than the second.

In relation to staffing we can start with the narrower definition and look at general practice. Table 3.1 shows the figures for England for selected years since 1973 in relation to independent GP principals, their list sizes and the size of partnership in which they were working. This shows the steady increase in the number of GPs and the consequent fall in the average size of their patient lists. The trend in terms of partnerships is also very clear. Larger partnerships have become steadily more usual although there remain a significant number of GPs practising single handed or in small groups. The figure for Assistants in general practice confirms the dominance of the concept of the full independent principal as the normal model of working, although of course locum practice is quite common. This means that the 1400 doctors training to be GPs at the time of writing would, if they enter practice on completion of their training, move immediately to become fully-fledged principals, with locum practice as the main intermediate role in which to develop their skills and knowledge further.

The change in partnership size is important, partly for its potential in relation to the way in which general practice itself can develop, but also because it carries broader implications in terms of organizing a wider scope of primary care. Before looking at that issue in more detail Table 3.2 shows the details of practice staff employed by GPs since 1984. This illustrates the scale of this aspect of primary care, but more importantly shows some key changes taking place more recently. The steady growth in the employment of practice nurses until they equate overall with one per practice in 1994, is of great importance although of course their distribution is not even across practices. In terms of support for practices the steady rise in computing staff since 1990 is significant, although it suggests that practices vary sharply in how far they have computerized and perhaps even more in the degree to which they have recognized the need for additional staffing to make more effective use of information technology. Or perhaps the growth reflects the narrower impact of fundholding where a specific need arises and where resources are more readily available to provide such support.

The other figure of interest is the growth in the number of practice managers though this must be read with caution in terms of what that role may involve. However it is indicative of an increasing recognition that there is a management role within general

Table 3.1 Numbers of GPs and practice sizes: selected years (England)

	1973		1983		1990		1994	
	No.	*%*	*No.*	*%*	*No.*	*%*	*No.*	*%*
Number of GPs	19,997		23,254		25,622		26,567	
Average list size	–		2,116		1,942		1,900	
Partners – Single	3,715	18.6	2,952	12.7	2,975	11.6	2,824	10.6
2 or 3	9,339	46.7	8,996	38.7	8,446	33.0	7,862	29.6
4 or 5	5,396	27.0	7,726	33.2	8,650	33.7	8,975	33.8
6 or more	1,547	7.7	3,580	15.4	5,551	21.7	6,906	26.0

Adapted from: Department of Health (1995b: Table 6.14).

Table 3.2 Staff employed by general practitioners 1984–94 (selected years)

	1984	1987	1990	1994
Total whole time equivalent	25,994	29,320	45,333	51,833
Practice managers	–	–	4,595	6,221
Computer operators	–	–	500	1,557
Secretary/receptionists	19,441	21,550	30,576	32,683
Dispensers	329	400	811	961
Nurses	1,924	2,768	7,738	9,099
Other	4,300	4,602	1,113	1,312
Ratio staff/GP principals	1.1/1	1.2/1	1.8/1	2.0/1

Note: Before 1990 practice managers and computer operators were listed under other staff.
Adapted from: Department of Health (1995: Table 6).

practices that can be carried by someone other than a GP partner (Huntington 1995). Certainly the evidence emerging from evaluation of fundholding where most work has been done, confirms the variety of people involved in practice management, but also confirms the significance of the role at least in relation to fundholding (Audit Commission 1996a).

Staying with general practice, other data indicate a wide pattern of variation though with some systematic flavour to its distribution. Doctor list size is not of course a direct guide to the quality, or character, of service, though conscious efforts have been made to reduce list size as though it was directly related to service quality. List sizes have in consequence fallen steadily from an average of 2116 in 1983, to 1900 in 1994. These figures hide a wide variation across the different regions of the country, currently ranging from 1692 in the south-west to 2026 in north-east Thames, with population density, and relative need, conditioning the impact of such variation. Inevitably such averages hide the detailed variation which at practice level runs from under 1000 to over 3000 patients per GP, posing at least a prima facie question about the work load and the relative character of care in such diverse cases. These figures are not here being seen in relation to indicators of need in practice populations, but they do affect the resourcing of each practice and as a result may also influence the pattern of provision over and above that offered by the GP.

Recognition that these variations are important was implicit in the early appointment within the NHS of the Medical Practices Committee (MPC). This was established to prevent doctors increasingly choosing the more desirable, and consequently overprovided areas, and as a consequence persuade some to set up in the less desirable urban centres. The implications for list sizes are obvious. This is reinforced by special allowances within the contract to compensate GPs for the demands inherent in practice in the less popular areas. In spite of this a study in the late 1980s examining regional financing and provision of family practitioner services concluded that there was 'considerable inequality in levels of finance and service provision which coincide with the existing inequalities of hospital and community services' (Birch and Maynard 1987: 538). More recently a direct examination of the distribution of GPs found what it called 'alarming inequalities' with the worst-off areas being in the North and the best-off areas in the South (Hacking 1996). This analysis at Family Health Service Authority (FHSA) level of course disguises the more local variations in both practices and health care needs which arise in specific, and often very needy sublocalities such as inner cities.

More particular evidence about practices is available now as a result of the work of the Audit Commission in looking principally at fundholding. This needs to be read against the fact that the scheme was not popular with all GPs, and that it was restricted to larger practices during its earlier phases. However, there may be some reason to suppose that fundholders would reflect the wider picture of general practice, particularly by 1995 when they involved one third of all practices and cared for almost half of all patients. A review of the scheme after five years of operation confirmed the diversity of practice, concluding that 'a few fundholding practices have achieved change in many of the areas listed. [The majority] have focused on achieving one or two significant gains for their patients' (Audit Commission 1996b). The detail of the report, reviewing service to patients (not direct clinical care of course) revealed wide disparities on all counts among the practices being reviewed. From the point of view of the wider general practice, it might be thought that fundholding would involve practices who would be at the more adaptive end of primary care development, but clearly variation is rife even among them.

Data from the reviews of fundholding are limited in relation to clinical care details, but do bear on the issues of comprehensiveness and coordination discussed earlier. Examination of relationships with other agencies, in secondary and community care, indicate a wide diversity of practice and of outcome. They do, however, suggest that the processes necessary to control and manage patient care in the new primary care-led NHS are slow to develop. The relationship with secondary care seems not fundamentally different to how it always was, and, with social services, remains underdeveloped. More significant perhaps is the increasing role played by the manager in those external contacts, with the GPs less involved as a result. This suggests either that the coordination role inherent in contract setting and monitoring is accepted as a managerial one, or that the formal aspects of the relationship are seen by GPs as less important than the informal relationship around individual episodes of patient care. These may not be changing as much as the theory of the quasi-market would suggest.

Of course, as has been pointed out earlier, primary care involves much more than general practice. General practices themselves employ an increasing range of other staff, extending the direct service that they can offer but also facilitating their ability to work with an even wider range of others within the community setting. This extended range of participants reinforces the case for a leading role for primary care, but adds greatly to its complexity.

Figures for 1993 show almost 38,000 primary health care nursing staff, a figure that has not altered greatly for some years, reflecting their long-standing role in primary care (Department of Health 1995c). Looking more closely this involves some 10,000 health visitors and 9000 district nurses. Examination of figures for activity reflect a dense pattern similar to that for general practice. In 1993–94 district nurses, community psychiatric nurses and community mental health nurses accounted together for 2.5 million initial contacts. These were dominated by district nurses but the scale of this very heavy work load confirms the significance of community nursing in relation to any overall view of primary care. Health visitors show an even larger figure with more than 3.5 million persons visited at home in 1993–94. Together these figures indicate the contribution of nursing staff to primary care, a view that is reinforced when the work is considered in relation to the concepts discussed earlier where accessibility and continuity of care were so important. The importance of home visits in this work, and the availability of longer periods of contact with patients are very significant.

Extending the discussion to social work is somewhat more difficult but in the context of debate about primary care it is important to do so. Local authority social services departments employ over 70,000 people in providing residential care, and about half that number again in managing and providing fieldwork services such as social work, occupational therapy and the like. If one adds the almost 60,000 who manage or provide domiciliary services then the scale of social service contribution is very obvious, as is the continuing character of a great deal of the support that they provide. Its overall professional content is more varied, but at the core in terms of primary care are a significant number of fully qualified social workers.

It is not part of the discussion here but the huge scale of informal care, all provided within the community setting, should not be forgotten. This is crucial to the pattern of demand for formal primary care services and ought to be taken into account in any strategic debate about the future of primary care.

CONCLUSIONS

This discussion has confirmed the complex character of primary care, both in terms of the way in which it is conceived, and of those whose professional role meets those criteria. It has also confirmed the strong dependence of those professional staff on a large number of informal carers, and a growing number of support staff of various kinds. The complexity of primary care evident in the summary details of practice across a range of services poses a strong challenge for a primary care-led NHS. It raises a number of issues in relation to the reforms already underway, and offers some prima facie argument for a wider consideration of reform despite the fatigue many already feel at the scope and pace of change.

4

SEEING CONNECTIONS: MODELS OF SYSTEMS

The review of the history, recent policy development and current structure of primary care within the NHS reveals a highly fragmented system of delivering care, continuing inequalities in people's health, and a recurrent failure to achieve apparently agreed goals despite periodic reform of the institutions of care. The most recent changes break with earlier approaches to reform and have adopted new strategies to deal with the legacies of the past. They have addressed the processes of policy making and the implementation of care delivery in new ways, and have adjusted the traditional structure in limited ways designed to meet the demands of the new market processes being introduced. In terms of the policy-making levels within the NHS this has produced a more streamlined and directly managed structure, but one that is highly centralized. In terms of service delivery it has increased the fragmentation by creating formally independent trusts and by introducing competition among providers and purchasers, enhancing divisions in the process. The requirements of the new NHS appear to work in opposition to one another rather than working together. Highly centralized targets and funding conflict with the concept of decentralized autonomy and decision making. Highly fragmented, independent and often competing, local provision conflicts with the need for strategies to be adopted which deal with the health needs of larger areas and with the overlaps of provision across the many service providers. This suggests the need for a reconsideration of the issues involved, which in turn suggests a need for much greater clarity about the characteristics of the NHS and what needs to be changed if successful reform is to be achieved.

A MODEL OF THE SYSTEM

One such approach has been widely applied in the examination of public policy particularly in the analogous context of urban government (Goldsmith 1980). This is the approach derived from systems analysis. A system is defined as a number of interactive elements which together make up a defined whole; analysis is concerned with how the whole system relates to its environment and how the elements within the system interact in doing so. The approach is essentially dynamic involving continuing mutual adaptation within both the system and the environment in response to their interactions.

Figure 4.1 presents a general model of government seen as such a system. It visualizes government as a system designed to deliver organized and authoritative decision making. The focus on government in this formal way deals with the problem of defining the boundaries of the system being analysed. By using the institutional

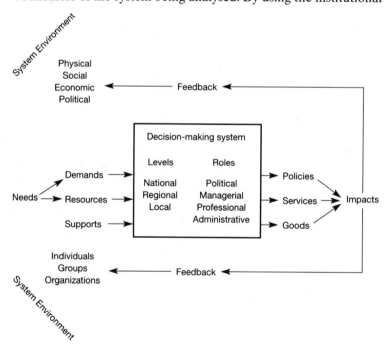

Figure 4.1. The basic system model

arrangements of government both the formal structures of decision and the geography of the relevant environment are defined. The system boundary is defined as an open one, allowing interaction with the environment through formal democratic procedures which legitimize decisions, and through informal contacts that provide the basis for decisions about whether or not to take authoritative action, and what action to take. The model sees the outputs from this decision-making process impacting on the environment, changing the character of future inputs into the political system from the environment and in turn producing further reaction. This cyclical process continues over time with mutual adjustment in both the environment and within the decision-making system.

This simple interactive model provides a useful way of conceptualizing the processes of government and certainly fits quite well with the description of policy development in the nineteenth century outlined in Chapter 1. It also provides a useful basis for examining the more recent changes in government and the NHS and a starting point for discussion about future development. Such extensive use of the ideas does of course require the approach to be further refined both in terms of the concept of the system environment and of the system itself.

Figure 4.1 does this with the environment conceived as involving two linked sets of elements. One involves the complex range of substantive factors relevant to the decision-making system including the physical, social, economic and political. The other involves the social structural elements which condition the political processes within the environment. Each of these elements may be conceived as acting independently on the system, and some parts of the system may be defined as having a formal concern with only one environmental aspect. The elements can also act together to produce more complex inputs which in turn engage the system in more complex ways as was evident in the discussion about nineteenth-century development in health policy. This substantive view of the environment does not take us very far, however, and we need some conceptual basis for understanding how and why some factors become relevant to government and others do not. This introduces the second environmental element and the figure illustrates a number of ways in which the linkages between the environment and the system may be conceived to give some shape to the processes involved.

At the most basic level, it suggests that environmental conditions generate needs that could in principle be met by government action, or are currently met by government but not always adequately or equitably. Needs in themselves do not impinge directly on systems, unless system rules have been established to regularize and automate responses to defined needs, as in the case of compulsory schooling, and even in such cases government action may vary widely in response. In relation to the model it is the translation of some needs into demands that converts them into inputs to the decision-making system, raising at least the possibility of response. Demands as inputs arise from situations in which some individual or group external to the system perceive that circumstances justify government action and articulate that need to those within the system. In the case of established systems, and the NHS is a good example, such demands may also arise from those who work within the system creating what are characterized as 'withinputs' in the literature (Easton 1965). The character and style of external demand varies with the nature of the external political and organizational processes involved and the power and influence of those making demands; similar factors apply to 'withinputs'. Successful demand depends on how these external (or internal) forces interact with the system and how the system is organized to process its response.

Need expressed as demand is not of course the only environmental consideration. System capacity to respond depends on other factors in the environment. Government willingness, and ability, to respond to demand is conditioned by two other environmental features: support and resource. Support reflects the degree to which the population concerned accord legitimacy and approval to the system in general, to the way in which it takes its decisions and to the particular policies and actions that it develops. In formal terms this may be provided periodically through elections, loosely mandating and legitimizing a range of actions. There are occasions however when situations generate concern and involvement outside that broadly legitimate scope, producing particular outcomes which may not accord with such mandated general policy. Such occasions create informal interactions that in turn may affect subsequent formal support.

Resources are the factor that allows policy to be converted into actions which can in their turn materially affect the environmental conditions that gave rise to demand in the first place. Only when resources are forthcoming and the political and economic costs of their use are acceptable, will action occur. The scope of that action will involve all these factors being called into play and will of course depend on how they are perceived and dealt with within the system.

Moving within the political system, Figure 4.1 shows an important distinction between the structures established within the system for taking decisions, and the processes which go on around those structures. Recognition of need within the system, and response to demands that are articulated depend on the way in which the political system is organized and the attitudes and relative influence of the participants working within the system. So too do decisions about the scale of resources to be used and, equally important, how they will be allocated to meet competing demands. In terms of the overall political system the structure is shown as involving different horizontal levels of decision, linked in formal ways with clear divisions in terms of power and responsibility, reflecting hierarchy within the system. It is also shown as involving similar vertical divisions, again defined in formal ways, reflecting sectors and divisions having formal responsibility for taking relevant decisions.

These formal structures provide the setting around which processes for decision making are organized. In part this involves the development of parallel informal structures, but both formal and informal are determined in their operation by the range of roles that characterize the process. Within the political system four roles predominate: political, professional, managerial and administrative. Each has its own formal contribution to make to the debate about policy and its conversion into action. Those formal roles combine in varied ways related to the character of the decision and the stage in the decision-making process, to the level in the formal hierarchy and the character of the sector or division involved. Role players are also involved in extensive informal networks of interaction which may influence decisions and, even more profoundly, influence action. Each role carries its own perspective on the desirability and the implications of policy and action, and each carries a different legitimacy and responsibility in terms of accountability for any responses made.

Government action therefore involves much more than the recognition or acceptance of need or indeed simple response to expressed demand. The politician must take a view about the desirability of raising resources to meet need and demand, while the professionals and managers will have views reflecting their different roles in the use of such resources to implement necessary action. Agreement about the action to convert political priorities is not automatic but a result of the interplay among these groups. Within government the managerial role and the administrative role are often intertwined, adding significantly to the difficulty in implementing the Conservative government's reforms with their emphasis on management. The results of this process vary. Where there is agreement, as is often the case in established areas of government action, then further action readily follows. Where there is conflict, delay in the formal recognition of need or response to demand is common, or it may be that formal recognition of the need for action is agreed, but the level of action taken is limited.

These system characteristics were clear in some of the earlier discussion reflecting the usefulness of the approach. Support for voluntary activity, permissive legislation, pilot experiments with possible future adoption of their results, partial approaches and the mediation of action through other agencies or local governments are devices that were often used in early periods of policy making. Such caution is often the perceived cost of political agreement to act at all where formal structures are not developed or where conflict is overt. Of course it may also result from the cost (tax) implications of wider action, especially for politicians, or the inability to know exactly what to do where innovation may be involved and professional roles and capacities are not fully developed. Once professionals have become involved within government then there is often an internal voice in favour of responding to demand, adding to the probability of positive response, though also sometimes conditioning the response to maintain traditional professional roles.

As a result a decision to take action by government may not at once imply acceptance of any particular goal, but in terms of the model it does mark the beginning of the interactive cyclical process outlined earlier. Modest beginnings have been the hallmark of government intervention. Over time, however, the impact of intervention on patterns of need and demand, the creation of capacity to take action, and the changing expectations of providers and consumers of services, tend towards acceptance of more elaborate goals. Achievement of those goals is a different matter. This depends on the nature of the need being met, the capacity to meet it, and the character and quality of the decision process, which have been shown to be highly complex. Achievement also depends on the role players involved. For politicians, the assertion of policy positions with their symbolic significance may be enough to maintain support and position. For professionals and managers, delivery of the service implied may be more significant and their legitimacy will depend as much on colleague perceptions as on the public response.

SUBSYSTEMS

So far we have discussed the model in terms of the general characteristics of the government system, but of course the reality is that government is organized in a highly fragmented way into a large number of interacting subsystems, each involving its own relevant environment and variant of the decision-making pattern. This fragmentation is particularly important in the case both of health care in general and primary care in particular. Figure 4.2 illustrates the complexity using just four of the subsystems with fairly clear relevance for health. Each of these subsystems responds to the substantive needs and the consequent demands arising from its environment, and its response is conditioned by the resources and supports that have developed and become relevant and legitimate to its own prime concerns. Reactions in the subsystems that are not directly involved with health sometimes mitigate and sometimes exacerbate the context for health care though rarely as a result of direct concern for such outcomes.

For example, few would doubt from the historical and contemporary evidence that housing conditions have a dramatic effect on people's health. Failures in the housing subsystem to deal satisfactorily with those conditions reflect the weakness of demand, the fluctuating politics of housing, and the economics involved in any more elaborate response. The consequences of this failure within housing of course creates enormous pressures on health care but the formal separation of the two systems maintains independent patterns of decision making unless they can be brought into closer

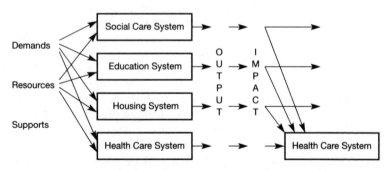

Figure 4.2. Model of subsystems

contact either at the operational level or more influentially at higher levels within government. The remedies available within the health care system reflect the character of that system and often involve a concentration on individual solutions, in sharp contrast to housing, where the nature of the system allows for a more collective approach to both need and demand. The mitigating effects of such action within health care are usually beneficial to the individual concerned, but may act to reduce demand for action within the housing subsystem, and in so doing may reduce the prospects for reducing health need more generally.

The same analysis could be offered in relation to other subsystems, and indeed the impact of health care decisions has its similar effect on the other related subsystems. Within government more broadly these issues of interaction between subsystems are recognized, as was shown in the earlier discussion. Failure to produce more satisfactory solutions is testimony to the complexity of the problem, but also more directly to the failure to address some of the difficult subsystem relationships in the reform process. The structure is so well entrenched that solutions are usually sought within the existing subsystems, with little institutional scope for looking across subsystems at more radical solutions.

THE HEALTH CARE SUBSYSTEM

Turning to the health care sub-system itself, Figure 4.3 illustrates the presence of further complexity within health care. It shows three related subsystems of health care formally operating within the NHS, and further divisions within these subsystems. The analysis of each such subsystem is no different from that which would apply at higher levels but their mix greatly complicates the service with important consequences for the health care, and health, of the society. Once again needs and demands vary across the subsystems with each reflecting a combination of both formal concerns and the development of informal patterns of service in the past. At this level of analysis, however, determination of need and demand are a combination of formal and informal requirements imposed from higher levels within the structure, and of local practice reflecting varied responses to those impositions. The higher levels become part of the environment for lower levels. Such local practice may reflect much clearer awareness of need and demand than is possible at higher levels within the NHS and will of course also reflect

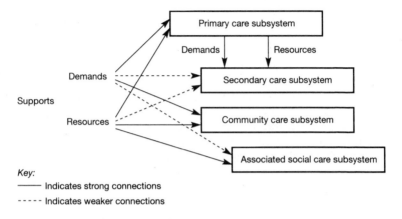

Figure 4.3 The health care system

horizontal relationships across the subsystems. This is complicated further by the fact that demand is formally filtered between subsystems, though with varied patterns of direct access also being available to complicate matters. The primary care subsystem provides extensive services, but also acts as the filter to secondary care and some community care, giving it great significance. This is conditioned by the fact that those subsystems also enjoy some direct access, evident in the increased use of accident and emergency services, and the extended first use being made of community nursing services.

Supports and resources are just as relevant at subsystem level as at higher ones within the service. A significant difference is that support tends to be derived from higher levels within the health care system so that it becomes a function of the formal and informal links that are put in place. The legitimizing formal political processes are national and the legitimacy of subsystems derives in part from that. There is also an informal support pattern evident locally as has been seen in the extensive conflicts generated whenever closure of hospitals is on the agenda. General acceptance of professional roles and the legitimacy of the controls which govern them provides a form of internal and external support for their operational activity, though it can be used more widely in conflicts over other issues.

Resource allocation is equally complicated and important, with the matching of effective demand with appropriate resources being critical to the future development of the NHS. Because of their political significance, control over aggregate resources is maintained in the politically sensitive central hierarchy. Demand on the other hand is a function of individual decisions taken at the other end of the spectrum and almost exclusively a matter of professional concern. Bringing demand and resource together is consequently difficult and the Conservative government's reforms have engaged new ways of doing so as was shown in Chapter 2. At present the allocation of resources remains complex, but is increasingly being managed through horizontal relationships at the subsystem level unlike the previous situation where allocations were made from the centre directly to each subsystem. The new structure gives some reality to the idea of a primary care-led NHS though the informal developments that are emerging around these structures already pose some questions about how the new approach will fare in the future.

The implications of these changes for the resource–demand equation may be judged from the fact that 90 per cent of encounters in the health service occur in primary care while 20 per cent of health care resources are used in that subsystem. Secondary care on the other hand receives almost 60 per cent of the resources to support provision of only 10 per cent of health care treatments. This inversion of demand and resource is of course partly explained by the relative cost of treatment in the two sectors of care. More importantly, the disparity reflects a varied response to patterns of demand, let alone to established patterns of need, but most closely reflects the long-standing patterns of organization and influence within the health care subsystems. The persistence of this inverse relation and the difficulty of reducing the imbalance between demand and resource allocation has been a recurrent theme as has been discussed, and yet the subsystem model has remained largely intact. Whether changing the dynamics of the subsystem relationships will assist the overall goals of equity and optimization remains to be seen.

Disparities between subsystems within the NHS are echoed again as one moves down the system towards the point of service delivery. Organizational arrangements within subsystems in their turn produce sub-subsystems in which decisions are taken about service and about the formalities of local service delivery. Conceptually, and in practice, these sub-subsystems operate as independent decision systems, reflecting their own patterns of need and demand, and having their own structures and processes for decision making.

Each is also affected by the actions of systems further up the health care hierarchy, and by those in parallel sub-subsystems. This complex pattern does not guarantee systemic uniformity, or compliance with higher levels of decision and one of its justifications is the need for sensitive response at this level. Wide differences result at the local level, between geographical areas and between practices in primary care, and between geographical areas, clinical specialisms and institutions in community and in secondary care. These are well understood and have been the object of government action over many years, without sufficient effect on ultimate allocations or outcomes to achieve Starfield's (1992) objectives. In fact the nature of the health subsystems has meant that in some cases one subsystem has been engaged in coping with the inadequacies of another, with relationships across their boundaries seldom reflecting rational approaches to overall health care. Current reforms have addressed the relationships between the elements in the overall system, but it may be that a more radical reform is indicated by a more self-conscious application of this analytic approach.

PROCESSES WITHIN SYSTEMS

These broad system and subsystem considerations provide some general pointers to structural factors which condition the successes and failures of public policy and service delivery. Equally important, as we have already observed, is the machinery for taking decisions and carrying them through within systems and subsystems. Analytically this is outlined in Figure 4.4, which distinguishes three key elements: structure, process and participants. The process element involves a set of rational assumptions about the way in which systems operate. Ideally the system responds to the pressures and possibilities from its environment by determining policies which in turn are followed by implementation into direct action. The relationship between policy and implementation varies according to a wide range of factors. Congruence between policy and practice is high where consensus about policy is well established, the character of the policy is clear, and practice well established (Alford 1969).

Where those features are not present then one expects looser policy frameworks, generous parameters allowing scope for diversity of acceptable practice, and highly permissive frameworks.

Level in the system	Roles played in the system			Agendas within the system		
	Political	Managerial	Professional	Policy	Resources	Implementation
National	****	**	*	***	***	*
Regional	*	**	*	*	*	*
Local	*	***	*	*	**	***
Sublocal		*	****		**	****

Note: The asterisks indicate the relative weighting of roles and agendas at the different levels within the system

Figure 4.4 Structure and process in the health care system

Medicine illustrates the tension in this model with policy often being made by politicians and civil servants, but clinical practice depending heavily on professional values. This has been acknowledged historically in the acceptance of clinical freedom subject to professional oversight, but policy clashes with such freedom when resource availability begins to dictate action. The politics of such a system are concerned with issues of compliance and are greatly affected by the structures established within each system but also by established patterns of relative influence among participants.

Throughout the British model this structure is complicated by the vertical sectoral division discussed earlier and also by the horizontal divisions that apply. In all public services there is a clear national arena where authoritative decisions are taken, which are processed through regional structures and implemented at a local, or in some cases, sublocal level. This structure does not conform directly with the division between policy and implementation, however, since both activities occur at each level. The mix does vary, however, moving in favour of implementation as one goes further down the system. Nor are policy and implementation confined within levels. National policy, unless purely symbolic, is most often implemented at other levels, and legitimate policy making at lower levels may conflict with national policy. The structure allows diverse influences to have effect on the processes of decision greatly influencing the congruence achieved between policy and implementation.

These diverse influences arise in the main from the activities of the key players in the process: politicians, professionals and managers, occupying authoritative or influential positions at all levels. Outcomes vary with the relative power and influence exercised by each group within the structure, and of course are affected by changes in structure and consequent changes in formal and informal relationships. In the case of health care, the reforms outlined in Chapter 2 have all affected those relationships, shifting power and influence between groups and changing the shape and location of the arenas in which they are exercised. Historically the system has sought to separate issues about priorities, resourcing and practice. Power over the clinical content of practice has legitimately been left with the professionals sustained by their professional organizations. Historically the professions have extended that legitimate power into strong influence on other areas such as resourcing and management, areas that are the legitimate domain of other groups within the system. One consequence has been the poor match between policy and practice, or intention and outcome, but another has been the very limited influence of managers and administrators within the system.

PRIMARY CARE

An understanding of this broad framework is essential to the main purpose here, which is to understand the primary care system and the changes necessary if the NHS is more closely to meet Starfield's (1992) objectives. This focus offers several advantages. Plans to redirect the NHS give a more significant role to primary care, making an understanding of how that system works, and of the process of intersystem relations, central to any radical programme of reform.

This is important because of the way in which the system and subsystem have developed over time. Structurally, general practice has always been organized outside the framework of the wider health care system, which itself was highly fragmented until recent years. Historically this was not a result of analysis of the needs of a health care system, but was a function of the political influence of doctors in general, and GPs in particular, which secured for the latter a formal status and contractual position outside the direct management of the NHS. This gave a particular shape to the relationship between primary care and secondary care, and between primary care and other parallel systems of care, within or on the fringes of the health care system. Much subsequent reform has been aimed at changing that situation with varied degrees of success.

In terms of working relationships the implications of these structural divisions were significant. As has been shown access to the health care system was through general practice with referral to other subsystems the basis of access to specialized care. The GP autonomy explicit in the structures of the health care system, and in the professionalization of medicine, easily spread into the operation of such cross-boundary decisions. GP awareness was high in relation to referral for secondary medical care, medical education for all doctors being dominated by experience in the secondary sector. GPs were much less aware in relation to other subsystems such as community services and wide areas of associated social care. In both cases autonomy meant that referral was highly individualized and sometimes quite idiosyncratic. The result has been highly diverse patterns of referral, with varying degrees of awareness about the suitability of a referral, and with consequently varied health outcomes.

CONCLUSIONS

This review of systems thinking in relation to the NHS and primary care suggests a basis both for considering the Conservative government's reforms and for suggesting alternative possibilities for the future if we are serious about goals for care that involve optimization and equity. It seems that the reforms rest on the application of principles derived from commercial models of the market, adapted to deal with the requirements of a public service, and one which remains free of charge at the point of consumption. The discussion around the systems approach suggests that the injection of formal market concepts, without significant change in other features of the system, may not produce the outcomes intended – at least, that is, the outcomes enshrined in the rhetoric of debate on all sides. The historical analysis confirms that rhetoric and reality have seldom come together, but if it is intended that they should we can use this analysis to good effect.

It suggests three factors that must form an integrated approach to reform, rather than the singular and fragmented approach applied in the past. First is the need to look again at structures with their profound significance for the way in which systems can be accessed and for the way in which they are constrained in their reactions. This necessary analysis applies at all levels within the NHS, given the significance of the linkages hierarchically between levels in the system, and horizontally between sectors and between agencies within sectors. Second is the need to look at those working within the system, at their knowledge, skills and attitudes and in consequence at their varying patterns of education and training in preparation for those roles. Roles properly vary, but the history of the NHS is marked by the informal extension of some roles into areas where their legitimacy may be called into question. They need redefining, and given the character of the reforms, there are new roles which need to be incorporated into the structures, especially those of managers whose functions are new to the system and whose impact has significance in terms of both politics and the professions.

The third concern provides a context for these other considerations. Despite the rhetoric that calls for health to be taken out of politics, or that claims that the quasi-market will achieve such a result, decisions about health and health care remain fundamentally political. Once the political decisions are clear then professional and managerial considerations come into play, and there is a place for a dialogue between these players in relation to both kinds of decision. Given the resource levels involved, and the significance of health and health care to the whole population, the importance of the NHS politically needs to be reasserted. But more is needed. How the politics of the NHS are organized, and how the public is involved in the quality and character of their health and health care are fundamental questions. The quality of service may be a matter for professionals, but who gets service and when and how they get that service, are matters of equal importance and should not be left only to professionals. These issues form the basis of the next chapters.

5

PROFESSIONAL DIVISIONS

Two central themes are emerging from the discussion so far in relation to a future primary care-led NHS. One concerns the place within it of a wide range of players, but particularly of professional, or professionalizing, staff. Another concerns the appropriate structures within which those players should operate to deliver primary care. The lessons of history, and of the systems model, confirm the significance of both and the importance of how they interact to respond to the changing environmental factors which are relevant to primary care.

The rhetoric behind the Conservative government's reforms has acknowledged these issues, but it is being argued here that the reform process and the reforms themselves are not best designed to deal adequately with the lessons of the past. The government view that the interests of service providers should not predominate in debates about reform, and that neither unions nor professions should dictate the pattern of a future NHS reflects a reaction to a past when the medical profession enjoyed considerable influence. This has resulted in the relative marginalization of the main medical establishment from the debate about reform, and has of course not allowed those other primary care staff groups, historically much more marginal anyway, to fulfil their wish to have a more central role in debate about reform. The impact of this is exaggerated by the fact that many of the reforms themselves give government a more direct role in relation to professional practice. The traditional extension of professional influence from a narrow to a wider focus has been inverted in this process with government being seen as moving to influence previously legitimate professional concerns. The danger is that those same professions are expected to implement the changes being introduced, and acceptance of the legitimacy of change is an important factor in securing appropriate compliance.

This becomes more obviously the case if primary care is to assume a greatly extended role. This will move the debate from the particular concerns of the medical profession, or with GPs within it, to one that involves a wide range of other staff, traditionally seen as 'semi-professional' in status, or as 'professions associated with medicine' (PAMs), designations that define their place in the existing system and inhibit their impact on the debate. For a long time these associated groups have been seeking professional status and the parity of consideration which they think would flow from that, an aspect of future relationships which will not go away just because doctors are wielding less influence in the wider debate. The risk is that in this situation, failure by doctors to maintain their formal dominance through influence in the wider debate may lead to a struggle to retain their position through the process of implementation.

This possibility assumes greater significance as the reforms in primary care carry development forward from the traditional model with the GP as the sole professional, to a position where a multiprofessional Primary Health Care Team (PHCT) is being acknowledged, to a future where interprofessional working will become the norm. These changes suggest an urgent need for a review of current professional education and training for primary care, with the possibility of a quite different pattern of professional education and organization in the future to meet the demands of the new NHS (Barr 1994).

Debate about the nature of the professions and their role in society has a long history (Wilding 1982). One strand of argument concerns those characteristics of an occupational group that give it a claim to 'professional status'. Another relates to the wider social, economic and political influence accorded to occupations that successfully establish their professional status. The characteristics which make for a profession normally include extended education and training prior to entering practice; a discrete body of learning forming the basis of that practice; controlled admission to, and removal from, professional practice; acceptance of ethical codes governing practice; but most importantly, all of these matters being determined and managed by the profession itself. For the individual, professional status brings a high level of working autonomy freed from non-professional constraints on what is done. For the profession as a whole, as we have seen, it has been used to extend that working autonomy to support a wider collective influence over the context in which professional work is undertaken.

Medicine is often cited as the ideal/typical example of such professionalization, while nursing and social work enjoy a lower 'semi-professional' status (Etzioni 1969). In all three cases, extensive education, training and experience supervised by established professionals precedes admission to the profession but only in the case of medicine does autonomous clinical practice formally follow from that preparation. The General Medical Council and the various Royal Colleges exercise the necessary organizational, ethical and practice controls that guarantee individual standards. Nursing and social work have more recently developed structures though the United Kingdom Central Council for nursing, and the Central Council for Education and Training in Social Work to play analogous roles. More importantly the employment structures for nurses and social workers give much more power to employing organizations than is the case for GPs who, being self-employed, are not so constrained and whose high level of individual autonomy in clinical practice is publicly accepted as legitimate because of professional controls. The logic of the medical case is clear. If effective practice requires particular knowledge, extensive training and close pre-practice supervision, then lay influence over its subsequent exercise is inappropriate. This raises obvious questions about why nursing and social work do not enjoy such autonomy and also how the managerialism, consumerism and market mechanisms being introduced into the NHS will affect this situation.

Historically this dilemma has not arisen because medicine successfully extended its professional influence into a wide array of non-clinical issues. As has been shown the organization of the health services has been decisively influenced in important respects by the medical profession. The profession have a legitimate interest in such matters, but their decisive impact cannot be justified on the same clinical grounds that underpin their professional standing. The same is true of resource allocation within the NHS. Disparities of resourcing between primary and secondary care, between different regions, and between different clinical specialisms are in part the resolution of competing professional interests within medicine. The profession has sought to speak with a singular voice when asserting its collective autonomy, but the exercise of that autonomy around the allocation of resources has reflected the pluralism and diversity of intraprofessional views and influence. Nursing and social work have never enjoyed such influence and indeed, in the case of nurses, have seen their roles greatly influenced by medical dominance within the NHS.

For all three professions, issues of status and legitimacy, with their impact on both practice and the way in which practice is organized, provide a key focus for the future. Current models of professional education and development will greatly influence the way in which they adjust to the changes being introduced into the NHS and to the implicit changes in their own relationships. This is given greater significance by the shift in the balance of power as government challenges the traditional autonomy of the medical profession both in general and in the more detailed practice of clinical care.

PROFESSIONAL EDUCATION – THE GENERAL MODEL

An obvious starting point for the necessary re-examination of this situation is the basic education that now governs access to the professions. In an extensive review of the professions Houle has provided a useful starting point (1980). Figure 5.1 adapts his general model of professional education for the three professions being considered in relation to primary care.

The key claim for professional expertise in the case of medicine derives from the scientific basis of medical practice with its explicit view of the causes of illness and the provision of appropriate treatment. This dictates that recruits into medical school are already

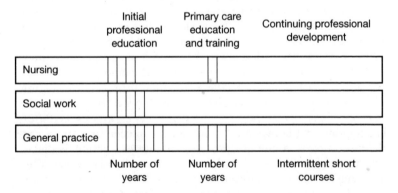

Figure 5.1 Professional education in primary care.
Adapted from: Houle (1980).

heavily specialized in science subjects at school and militates against mature students entering in most cases. Once recruited into medical school, that specialization is reinforced by three years of pre-clinical science. This extended specialized study provides the base for formal training in the skills of medicine through supervised experience of clinical practice on hospital wards and includes a very brief exposure to general practice. This training is followed up by further experience in hospitals refining what has been learned and developing through working alongside, and supervised by, established doctors practising established medical specialisms. Little of this experience is offered outside hospitals. Most experience is with very sick patients, rarely with the mildly ill or the chronically sick. Scientific method and hospital process together define the learning experience. Consultants and other senior doctors teach and junior doctors learn, ostensibly to become consultants in due course themselves.

Nursing and social work show some equivalence to this model but the pattern of development differs in important ways. In the case of nursing, unlike medicine, there are several entry routes and patterns of initial professional education leading to different careers in practice. Pre-entry standards are less demanding in general than those in medicine, in terms of both the subjects seen as necessary for entry and the standards expected of student applicants. This general picture has been changed by the advent of undergraduate courses in nursing, which reflect higher levels of entry often analogous to medical school. The content of education is broader than for medicine though the basic science is similar, and the much shorter training period is seen as implying a lower level of development. As with medicine there has been a strong tradition of extensive supervised practical experience on hospital wards reflecting the emphasis on skill development within the profession.

Social work is different again though there are some similarities with both of the other models. Like nursing it involves several levels of entry, related to the varied levels of professional status within the occupation. Background subjects necessary for entry are drawn from the social sciences, with their different intellectual criteria, and more importantly are subjects that do not find such a prominent and established place in the school curriculum. This opens the way for later entrants whose life-experiences are often deemed to be as important as their more formal education, with obvious implications for the traditional justification for professional status. Once into formal preparation, however, the process follows a similar pattern, with relevant subjects taught at degree level and experience gained under supervision in the field.

In short all three occupations, in part at least, follow the traditional professional model. The variants of background, timing and character of the initial process are followed by quite different patterns of development which greatly affects how each profession is perceived. This makes the post-qualification experience important. In the medical case the end goal is independent practice, universally in the case of general practice, though within hospitals there is a varied period of formal supervision until a consultant post is achieved. In nursing and social work the picture is more complex. Formally, both are occupations in which supervision of practice is a continuing feature throughout the whole career. In many situations of course the provision of supervision is not always straightforward and the character and quality of supervision can vary widely. Whatever the reality, the formal requirement inhibits nursing and social work from enjoying the full status of professionals, but of course the practicalities of work, especially in detached community settings, allows them to enjoy much the same autonomy as doctors do.

TRAINING FOR PRIMARY CARE

The character of the three professions merits further consideration, particularly in the context of an elaborated model of primary care. Social work prepares people for work in community settings as part of the basic system of training while medicine and nursing provide post-qualifying courses for those intending to work in primary care. Vocational training for general practice has a long history and has been compulsory for more than 20 years, with intending GPs required to undertake three years of formal training. This training recognizes the different needs of general practice and begins to compensate for the emphasis on hospital care in initial medical training, but the fact that two years are spent in hospital posts and only one year in general practice continues the dominance of the hospital tradition. The Royal College of General Practitioners (RCGP) have argued that five years are needed for a proper conversion to general practice, and there are current discussions, and some developments, introducing higher professional training to provide voluntary extensions to vocational training (Pietroni 1991; Smith 1994). Clearly the costs of five years would be considerable, and the alternative strategy of reducing the period spent in hospital would affect service provision in a dramatic way so that development on a broad front seems unlikely.

The problem with the current model stems from a number of sources. One is the search for a pattern of training which will equate to that of the established medical specialties in hospitals, despite the very different work for which GPs are being prepared. Another is that the creation of undergraduate departments of general practice has not greatly shifted the emphasis of initial training, so that reorientation is more difficult than it might be. This is reinforced by the fact that the move to general practice is seen as involving a move from team-based care to individual care, requiring a capacity to work alone on the part of the intending GP. This in its turn is reinforced by the system of training which does involve registrars working in approved training practices, but makes individual trainers formally responsible for training and approving the competence of individual registrars. Together these factors probably account for the emphasis on training GPs who are safe to practice, with summative assessment now confirming that emphasis on basic capacity rather than widening the focus and promoting excellence as the goal (Johnson *et al.* 1996a, 1996b). The content of training reflects the same emphasis with clinical skills dominant, and with limited attention paid to those wider concerns that might be relevant to the new doctor in the new primary care.

In these respects nursing and social work may have a better model, or one more suited to the demands of the future. Their initial training is shorter but in the case of nursing is followed by as much focused specialist training for community nursing roles as is experienced by GPs. Courses are provided, usually of one year's length to prepare nurses for the move from secondary care into one or other of the community nursing specialisms discussed in Chapter 3. These courses provide relevant studies in subject areas that are less usual in initial nursing but highly relevant to community based work, such as sociology and social administration. They also provide supervised practice in appropriate community settings. Practice Nurses are exceptions; they currently have little dedicated preparation, although some courses are developing and many will have worked in the community in one or other of the community nursing specialisms. In terms of primary care this may suggest rather more equal levels of competence than are suggested by the secondary care model where doctors enjoy much longer and higher level preparatory training. Levels of knowledge and skill are clearly related to the length of training, but the relevance of initial training to primary care work is limited by it being learned in the wrong context. Of course the relevance of early training may be more obvious in nursing given the practical nursing skills that may be involved in primary care, though the professional claims for community nursing rest on the argument that it involves much more than those traditional practical skills.

Social work is different again in that the basic training is a preparation for work in the community setting. Once again relevance becomes a central issue together with perceptions of that relevance across the professions. Social work has often been perceived by others as working to provide practical supports of various kinds, and much referral has traditionally reflected that view. Resource constraints within social service departments have sometimes made this an accurate perception, and of course the demands made by inappropriate referrals greatly inhibits the ability to practice other skills. This simply confirms the need for greater mutual awareness so the professional claims of social workers to provide a much more complex range of care and support may be acknowledged and brought into play.

LIMITS OF THE MODELS

Each of these models of professional training sits firmly within the traditions of the three professions involved and none of them has been driven by the changed context provided by the emerging models of primary care practice, let alone with the demands of the reformed primary care-led NHS. This is reflected both in the content of what is taught and learned and in the style and character of the educational process. Each profession caters adequately for the basic skills involved in its traditional practice, but much less so for the extended roles and changing demands that professionals face in the new system. Adaptability and flexibility are key attributes for the future of each profession and have been notably missing in some professional reaction to development in the past and in the reaction, again of some, to the more recent volatility in the NHS and social welfare generally.

Houle confirms the importance of this in his suggestions about a more appropriate model of professional development (1980). He suggests two recurrent needs in all professional careers, needs that have to be seen in relation to careers which extend over a 35-year period. One is the need to prepare for a range of new tasks that will inevitably arise in the context of any professional role, and the other the need for organized preparatory training and education before such roles are undertaken, if they are to be undertaken effectively. Both needs seem relevant to all the professions involved with the current developments in primary care, though the reform process seems not to have catered for either of them to be met. This may reflect the Conservative government view that the market, and its associated institutions, will dictate behavioural change and that the professions will simply adapt. Or it may reflect their acceptance of the fact that education and training are matters for the appropriate profession which must be left to reform their own systems to meet the new challenges. Or it may simply be a matter of cost. At the time of writing, the most recent government proposals seek to stimulate initiatives in this area working with the key interests involved in professional education (Secretary of State 1996c).

Seen against such needs professional training for general practice, social work and nursing share the same characteristics. Each highlights one hallmark of professional education, which is that the skills are learned at the outset of a career and from then onwards have to be sustained and refined by experience. This may have been adequate when the context of practice, and practice itself, were relatively stable, but in the much more volatile current climate experience may be a much less useful guide and may inhibit both innovation in practice and its adoption more widely in the professions.

All three professions share a further characteristic which is that formal continuing professional education is severely limited. Of course professionals have many ways of keeping up to date through reading, through research, through audit of their work, and through contact with colleagues, and more recently through the development of much more self-conscious 'reflective practice' (Schön 1983). Good though these approaches are, they are not universal, and some are not even commonly used, but all are inhibited by aspects of the current structures of practice. Many GPs are relatively isolated and work in an individualistic culture which inhibits some of these approaches. Nurses and social workers operate in environments that are not dominated by their professional cultures, but by the requirements of organizational and political imperatives that dictate much of their practice. The limits of self-directed development in all of these settings is very evident.

Formal continuing professional education might help to overcome such barriers. GPs have a system for this built into their normal activity and recognized in their formal method of payment. The Postgraduate Education Allowance (PGEA) was introduced in 1990 and funded by withdrawing the money from seniority payments and providing a payment to all GPs who attend up to 30 hours per year of formally approved education. The rules of this system provide for three categories of substantive concern, clinical knowledge, health promotion and practice management. Since the early 1990s there have been GP Tutors appointed on a part-time basis to oversee the operation of the system, approve content and seek to develop provision to reflect the changing needs of practice.

Social workers and nurses enjoy no such relative luxury and rely on employers funding occasional courses, or on their own capacity to continue their development while working in situations not resourced to accommodate continuing education. Resource limitations and the conflict between spending on training and on service greatly inhibit what can be done. The different professional situations of course limit the opportunities for interprofessional training as well, reinforcing patterns from the past.

In any case, compared to initial education, formal continuing education is infinitessimal in scale, and in the case of general practice a good deal of attention is directed at clinical areas familiar from initial education in medical school. The educational approach seems to be based on the view that medicine changes only a little throughout a career, that consultants and long-established GPs are simply very experienced doctors in their field, and that hospital and general practice careers do not change significantly with experience and seniority. Such a view seems to be manifestly wrong, but so too does the alternative explanation – that initial medical training equips the doctor to undertake any role that may crop up during a long career.

Two issues arise. One concerns the character of the professional career and the expectations that appear as careers develop in a changing context that has implications for what knowledge and skills may be required of professionals in primary care. The other concerns the implications of this concept of career both for initial professional education and training and for continuing professional education in its turn.

CAREERS IN PRIMARY CARE

As has been shown the three professions vary somewhat in their systems of education and training but medicine and nursing are alike in that primary care enjoys quite limited time relative to other aspects of their training. All three professions hold narrow views about what primary care involves, restricting their vision to the roles and relationships that have operated traditionally. The implications of this were evident in earlier discussion of the fragmented development of primary care and seem likely to become even more significant in relation to the wish for a more integrated approach in the future.

In terms of past experience professional training has little regard for how professional careers have developed and will develop. It provides poor preparation for the extended activities of GPs as they settle into practice and take on new roles within and outside their practices. It provides no preparation for nurses and social workers whose careers tend to 'progress' by leaving practice to take up supervisory or managerial roles which make quite different demands on them. In terms of the future, professional training as yet pays little regard to the multidisciplinary character of primary care or to the changing roles that might be played within it by each of the professions. Nor does it obviously prepare people for new roles that arise in the context of a central role for primary care in the development of the NHS.

This is not to suggest that the core of basic professional training leading to competent practice is unnecessary. It is to suggest that by itself it is not enough and that initial education and training need to reflect the fact that careers in primary care will unfold in varied ways and at varied speeds. The social and economic context of practice and, in particular, of patient need will vary widely and will change. The number and range of staff involved and the nature of their employment and contractual positions will also vary and again will change over time. In general practice, the number of partners, the pattern of financial rewards and different personal interests of those involved all dictate variation. Wider changes in the NHS, and the latest proposals for primary care, suggest that all of these factors may themselves change so that adaptation and adjustment become important skills for the future primary care professional whether doctor, nurse or social worker (Secretary of State 1996c). Initial professional education needs to prepare for this reality and for continuing professional education to reflect both that initial change and the moving context of primary care.

Figure 5.2 follows Houle but goes further in specifying several aspects of developed primary care practice which may be expected to form part of developing careers in the professions involved.

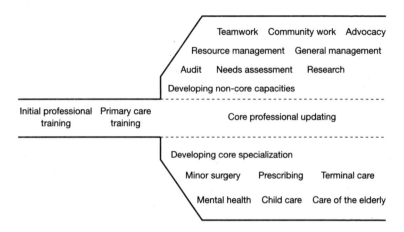

Figure 5.2 The developing primary care career

These differ somewhat between the professions, and of course individual careers will not develop in uniform ways. What is clear is that collectively the professions will have to cater for these areas of development if primary care is itself to develop and if its leading role within the NHS is to be realized.

First and foremost, given the backgrounds of the three professions, and the continuation of core activity, is the need for updating in relation to professional knowledge and skills together with the opportunity for possible specialization within the core professional role. In the case of medicine this may involve developing clinical specialization within the community setting (minor surgery, dermatology, asthma, paediatrics) or refining those clinical skills that are particular to general practice. The same may be true for nursing as community nurses take on extended roles, providing first contact care, prescribing, or dealing with health education programmes. For social work a closer association with primary health care could give rise to a range of developments, and even within the present arrangements the extended role in care management in community care is already apparent. Such developments will, by their character, not involve all professionals, but all professionals would benefit from basic grounding during their early education to extend their capacity for, and choice of, some of these possible specializations.

The corollary of developments such as these is the demand for a more coherent approach to the creation of primary health care teams who together have the specialist skills to deliver the pattern of community based care expected in the future. The teamwork essential to the practice of such specialization, and the management implications for primary care, will of course also have to be taken into account. In traditional general practice, management, such as it was, usually fell to the senior partner in a partnership. This was a satisfactory system given the limitations of practice, but the advent of fundholding and the considerable changes in general practice staffing have placed strains on that system. In some cases these have been met with the introduction of a role of executive (or fund-holding) partner which has not always gone with seniority. It may reflect an interest in developing that role on the part of another partner, and may reflect some training or expertise, but in the main there is little formal preparation for such roles. Performance in the role clearly depends on awareness of, and a capacity to deal with, organizational and management issues within general practice. These now go well beyond the traditional problems that arose in partnerships. Resource levels involved are often very high, allocation of such resources both visible and politically relevant, while staffing patterns are much broader than before and relationships outside practices are becoming more complex. The advent of specialist practice managers suggests that model is changing. In future the professional role in medical management may lie not in a GP directly managing, but in one or all GPs in a practice providing a clear input about the clinical and related professional needs of practice with a professional manager translating those into action. The necessity for all doctors to develop new awareness and skills remains. Such a managed model requires substantial change. For professionals used to autonomy, recognition of the need to be managed, and acceptance of the implications of being managed, will require changes in attitudes and the development of appropriate skills. Future managers may include GPs but the possibility of management being a marginal function fitted in alongside continuing practice seems unlikely.

Nursing and social work operate within a quite different tradition. In both, the career does not lie in a lifetime of professional practice, but often in promotion out of the professional role into a supervisory or a management position. The knowledge, skills and attitude for such roles are not inherent in the original professional training, and many enter managerial posts with little preparation beyond having been managed. This is much more acute than in the general practice case. In these professions management is seen as an essential aspect of the service and patterns of accountability in nursing and social work place much greater emphasis on the managerial role. The exercise of that role is greatly influenced by the fact that managers are drawn from the profession, and this sometimes gives rise to problems when the absence of preparation for management results in management being seen as a particular form of social case-work or a reflection of traditional relationships in nursing.

All three professions pose a problem in this context, which is pointed up by the development of managerialism within the wider NHS where the concept of general management holds much more sway, most obviously within secondary care. Even there, however, the clinical director has emerged, somewhat analogous to the executive partner or the managing nurse or social worker. The underlying principle in all these cases appears to stem from the argument that the professionals can only be managed by those who have practised, or in some cases it is argued, by those who continue to practise. The skills and attitudes involved in management, and the extent of the management role in complex organizations which interact widely with others, raises questions about that view. It may no longer be consistent to maintain the traditional position. Professional general managers will need to be sensitive to the proper scope of professional practice, but professionals in turn will need to recognize the demands of management in conditioning their practice. The relationship with management is no different in this respect from that which affects other interprofessional working.

A third role around the interface with other sectors of care had a limited place in the old system but has become central to the purchaser/provider split within the internal market in the NHS. Traditionally this has been a role for the GP acting as gatekeeper and exercising control over the system of referral and follow-up. Under the new arrangements it has become more formalized and enshrined in contracting processes, whether through fundholding or through other local purchasing arrangements. In such a context and with extended primary care teams there is of course scope for all the professions to play a role in the process, each bringing a perspective on need arising from their local knowledge. As with practice management, this need not necessarily involve the doctor in a direct role. Whether a fundholder, or involved in a district purchasing system, the doctor is the person who understands the clinical issues and patient interests that should lie at the heart of the market process but may not be the person to engage the contracting process itself. It is not merely a matter of clinical knowledge. Doctors may need to develop the skills necessary to communicate their clinical concerns to others operating directly in the market place. Mutual awareness and understanding are key ingredients in this complex process. As with other aspects of this proposed model, the tradition of autonomous practice, and the autonomous practitioner, will have to be overcome. The doctor need not do everything, or be able to do everything, but must be aware enough to secure that others take account of those needs which only doctors can understand. The same arguments apply to the other primary care professions, although their different past experiences may make the transition easier to make.

This characteristic also applies within two other areas of obvious concern in the future: community action and the primary care team. These are coupled together as both involve team working with a wide, though varied, range of other professions, and in both cases to some degree, with patients, and with the wider public. The relevance to primary care of many other professions, from the obvious health visitors and district nurses, to the less obvious teachers and community workers, needs to be understood. Implicit in such understanding is the need to develop the necessary knowledge and skills to work with those other professions. Such working probably cannot be reconciled with the old model of autonomous practice, and certainly is not consistent with a view of medicine as necessarily the most important contributor to health care in the community. This has been evident in the context of individual cases where the case conference has long recognized the professional linkages. It is the generalization of that view into everyday working and into policy development that seems important for the future.

Finally there is a realm of professional activity where experience may be developed in the service of other GPs, nurses or social workers and of the profession as a whole. This may involve roles within the representative structures of the profession through the British Medical Association or the Royal College of Nursing, or on a different level, activity in the RCGP or relevant professional body. It may alternatively involve a role in the vocational training system or in the development of continuing professional education for the relevant profession. It may come to include a wider range of new activities if the systems of the internal market become focused on consortia in which there is a need for individuals to represent the professional view in relation to a range of activities. These latter settings may be where the professional role and a possible market role overlap. They may also be the context in which the role extends further and involves the GP, nurse or social worker representing the patients as advocate, demanding new skills both in relating to patients as a group and also to other agencies and professional groups.

CONCLUSIONS

It is clear that the implications of a new model of primary care, and one that plays a much more self-conscious part in leading the NHS, raise important questions for the professions involved and for those designing and providing their education and training. The current models of professional training are closely linked to the practice of an earlier period and their fragmentation across primary care echoes the other divisions that inhibit development around the new models. The need for a re-examination of the system of providing education and training seems obvious.

6

ORGANIZATION AND MANAGEMENT

Earlier chapters have charted the emergence of different elements of the extended primary care system since the turn of the century, and have shown how resistant to change many aspects of the system have been. Reforms have taken place in the NHS at regular intervals, but have been mainly confined to intermediate levels of decision making, leaving the local service delivery subsystems relatively unchanged. Local government has also experienced reform, but this has focused on the relationship between central and local government, leaving the style and character of most service delivery much as it has always been. This has been particularly true for social services, which have not in any case been at the centre of the reform debate in local government.

The result is that each aspect of primary care is organized in a different way. Each reflects its different historical origins, the continuing power and influence of the key interests involved in provision, and the inertia that these forces create when the details of reform are being considered. Repeated suggestions for more fundamental change, most notably the idea of moving health care services into local government, have been aired repeatedly during the reform process but have always foundered on the opposition of the medical profession. In the case of general practice that professional opinion was allowed to influence the organization of service delivery, in part to secure GP compliance with development of any kind, resulting in quite modest degrees of change. Community health services have not been marked by such professional influence with the result that their structures are quite different with significant implications for practice and for possible relationships with general practice. Local government has been reformed, and social services experienced considerable upheaval after the

Seebohm Report (Seebohm Committee on Local Authority and Allied Social Services 1968), and their subsequent involvement in the more corporate management of local authorities. What the different organizations in these services do not reflect, and indeed were not designed to do so, are the needs of a modern integrated primary care system that can take a leading role in the development of the NHS.

This has become more important in the climate of the 1990s when the dialogue about health care and about the role of government has changed so that growth is no longer automatic and economic pressures make arguments about efficiency as important as those about distribution and about equity. As was shown in Chapter 2 this change of emphasis has produced significant changes in the framework within which local organizations operate, but no significant effort has been made to alter those organizations themselves. Discussion of the systems model in Chapter 4 suggested that changes in environmental opportunities and constraints and intersystem relationships brought by the internal market will change behaviour and decisions. It also suggested that without parallel changes in the structures of organization involved there might be a limit to the degree of change that could take place. Changed practice will result, and already has done so in some cases, with new relationships developing and in some cases with a reorganization of some care delivery. This seems to reflect, as one would expect given the model of reform and the evidence of past practice, the willingness of the innovatory few, and at some stage it is likely that voluntary changes will have to be codified into new and more widely applicable practices if radical outcomes are to be delivered. This is especially true if the goals being sought are ones that involve greater equity and more accountability across the system.

The argument advanced here is that the current reforms have tackled some of the elements that needed to be tackled, but that they have not gone far enough in addressing the need for reform. At least, that is the argument if the goals of reform do remain optimal provision and equitable access to health and health care.

THE CURRENT POSITION

If we take the current position in relation to the extended primary health care model and the Conservative government's intentions for the NHS then the difficulties become immediately apparent.

There are three quite distinct forms of organization and management involved with care delivery and much variation within each of those. The formal and informal arrangements that link these local delivery systems with national policy making also differ and are also complex. Despite this complexity, the new-style primary care depends on the systems working together to achieve broad national policy goals, and doing so with limited resources, with both central policy and resource allocation subject to regular changes in both the short and medium term. The difficulty of achieving integration between policy and implementation is widely acknowledged and various efforts are being made to secure local compliance.

One attempt is for policy directives to be framed more precisely and for national priorities to be made more explicit and public. *The Health of the Nation* (Secretary of State for Health 1992) targets, and the requirements written into the *Patient's Charter* (Department of Health 1995b), both illustrate that tendency and confirm the character of the Conservative government's national priorities. The targets initially concentrate on five key areas of priority: coronary heart disease and stroke; cancers; mental illness; HIV/AIDS and sexual health; and accidents (Secretary of State for Health 1992). The Charter involves a range of visible, but not directly clinical, aspects of the care process like rights to registration with a GP, health checks, and appropriate referrals and prescriptions (Department of Health 1995b). Further developments, and charters specific to each general practice, are being developed with emphasis placed on the care process and waiting lists and waiting times involved. In secondary care the publication of performance league tables in relation to such criteria is designed to provide a basis for decisions about referral on the part of health authorities and GP fundholders though coincidentally it also influences the internal priorities of hospital trusts. In primary care financial allocations are associated with the achievement of some of *The Health of the Nation* targets as in the case of immunizations and the initial health promotion targets. This approach is extended in the latest proposals for primary care development, which involve a search for performance indicators for general practice (Secretary of State 1996c).

These changes reflect the introduction of the market philosophy into the NHS and the need to provide some basis on which purchasers and providers can take decisions in a market that does not have a conventional cash and consumer basis. Patterns of mutual influence are changing as a result and, in theory at least, moving the stimulus for action closer to patients. The efficacy of these changes is of course conditioned by the levels of resource available, which constrain the targets being set, and the capacity of the system to respond. In a tight economic climate the targets and charter terms tend to direct spending and leave little capacity to redistribute resources both between and within sectors, which is one of the necessary aspects of the move to a primary care-led NHS. This limitation seems less relevant in the national context because of the central assumption that efficiency gains can be made in all sectors, including primary care, in order to facilitate new activity. The existence of explicit targets, and the implications of assumptions about resources, make organizational issues within primary care more significant, promoting an emphasis on interorganizational relationships and joint working as the key to success. Examination of the current forms of organization and management may throw some light on the possibility of such changes, and also suggest other reforms that may be needed.

GENERAL PRACTICE

Traditional primary care, in the form of general practice, seems relatively easy to describe, often being seen as little more than minor variations on the established model of the independent single professional practitioner. Chapter 3 illustrated how that model has changed since the early 1970s with single-handed practice giving way to group practice as the dominant pattern. In some cases of course group practice means little more than several independent practitioners working from the same premises and sharing limited joint services. Increasingly, however, it has come to mean much more for many practices though considerable variety of practice still remains within group practice. Practice partnerships involve shared concerns about jointly owned premises and about jointly employed staff. Wider resource issues also arise, and increasingly team working is becoming significant, but the core model of individual practice remains relatively intact in many cases both in form and in reality.

Many of the shared concerns arise from the fact that general practice involves self-employed doctors, so that practices, of whatever size, are in fact small businesses that share many characteristics with small businesses in any other sector of economic activity. Issues arise in relation to practice income, and individual GP income, but also about investment for the future in premises and in other aspects of care provision. These can all be complex, but pose particular dilemmas in a service funded directly from the public purse and one in which many aspects of the business are largely or entirely paid for by the state. Important issues about responsibility and accountability arise from this situation. At the same time this structure can make the reconciliation of particular practice goals with the wider goals for primary care within an area problematic. It is hard to find comparisons in other areas of professional life from which to draw ideas. Analogous models of organization can be found within accountancy and the law, but they have a much narrower client base, are funded by client fees, except for legal aid with its obvious problems, and their work does not constitute an essential public service like health care.

Some would argue that the concept of organization is barely relevant in the case of single-handed practice and a few might believe that it is not significantly different in the context of group practice. That view is challenged by the recent changes in the character of general practice and those that look likely in the future. Group practice, and fundholding in particular, have extended the number of staff involved; more recently, as was shown in Chapter 3, the type of staff involved has begun to change. Those changes have been reinforced by other changes, in levels of resourcing, in performance targets for activity, in demands for greater sensitivity to local health care needs, and an extended strategic role in relation to the wider NHS.

Support staff such as receptionists remain significant, but the widening workload has brought wider professional attachments in the shape of practice nurses, the occasional social worker, and increasingly consultants offering sessions and quasi-medical psychologists or counsellors are becoming more common within practices. Organizationally this has done much more than simply enlarge the team, although that itself poses problems. It has also changed the relationships among those involved from employer–employee, to co-professionals, some of whom are formally employed elsewhere with all the ties and controls which that can involve. This has increased the complexity of general practice, raising new issues about the allocation of work and how that should be decided, the channels of accountability between practice, profession and other employers, the supervision of quality and the allocation of resources to support practice. It is not yet clear how these extended organizations are coping with these features. In some cases the extended team may be handled as little more than a continuation of the traditional referral role of the GP, simply bringing more elements of the referred service within the practice. In other cases, serious efforts at teamwork, with shared decision making and flexible working are being tried. Certainly the shift from interorganization to intraorganization relationships changes their nature, and offers wide opportunities for further development as relationships mature and professional and patient experience changes. The ability to take advantage of these will depend on professional issues discussed in Chapter 5, but also on further organizational changes creating a more effective context in which development can take place.

Such changes are significant because they directly challenge the traditional patterns of power and influence in general practice. The model of GP control is inevitable in the narrow context of single-handed practice, but becomes much more complex in an extended practice setting. The formal employment status of staff becomes relevant here as this gives authority to the employer who in many cases remains the GP. Where this is not the case there is scope for conflict to arise about what is done and how it is done. It is worth remembering that the history of the NHS is marked by a recognition among GPs of the significance of their own employment status for their professional autonomy and their successful defence of their independent status. It is the recognition of that analysis in relation to other professions with whom they might work that lies behind the challenges posed by the current reforms in general practice.

These features of individual practice also have to be seen in the context of the sector as a whole. Most importantly, in terms of the targets of optimization and equity, this is a structure that makes for a high probability that variations will occur in the mode of operation, and the consequent character and quality of service offered by general practice. Greater consistency across the many practices involved depends in part on the uniform national systems of control exercised through common targets and formula funding. It also requires action at an intermediate level to oversee the work of practices and to filter the resources centrally allocated. Traditionally this involved little more than formal maintenance of contracts with the old Executive Councils who played little part in the broader aspects of practice development. The advent of Family Health Service Authorities (FHSAs) brought the start of a more active partnership in the development of primary care and the merger of FHSAs with health authorities (HAs) has provided a further stimulus to that role. This poses a challenge to the tradition of practice autonomy and places a heavy burden on managerial staff in the health authorities in handling delicate relationships with traditionally autonomous professionals. This is exaggerated by the fact that staff within health authorities have grown up with a different role in a different context, and the transition for them may be a very difficult one. The implications for practice organization and the ethos of professional domination pose sharp challenges. Professional direction remains established within the structure of the profession, which creates a national context for education and training and provides advice and advocacy about standards and about practice. This has to be reconciled with the new model of a managed, multiprofessional system if the reforms are to work.

This problem is reinforced by the nature of the clientele for primary care who form the other element in the organization of care. Unlike most professional organizations who provide episodic care to their clients, general practice is organized around a relatively stable register of patients; the terminology and the concepts about the nature of primary care discussed in Chapter 3 confirm this special character. Patients can of course change their practice registration, but this is a limited occurrence and the resulting monopoly position of the GP service provider influences the relationship with patients at any rate when they are considered collectively. This emphasis on patient choice, enshrined in the *Patient's Charter* (Department of Health 1995b), confirms the existence of their right to exit from a practice if dissatisfied, but the same charter also encourages the use of voice by patients as a way of influencing the quality of care within their practice (Hirschman 1970). This has always applied at the individual level, though patient take-up has been limited, but there has been even more limited experience of patients enjoying a collective say in how their practice is organized. The impact of this is reinforced by the nature of the clinical service, which creates a clear asymmetry in the power distribution between patient and doctor. Freedom from charges at the point of service reinforces this and the real benefits that follow in terms of access to care may be offset by some loss of patient legitimacy when seeking to influence practice policy. Inevitably it is the state funding mechanisms and controls, and the professional models of good practice, that mainly condition activity. The formulas for funding through capitation militate against patient influence in the main, though payments introduced with the 1990 contract to reward service performance have directed activity to some degree by making patient compliance more significant to some aspects of income, perhaps raising their potential influence. The system of funding provides a complex mixture of inducements and controls giving central government some control over activity in general practice, and channelled through the HA providing them also with an opportunity to influence practices.

Primary care in this sense thus lies at the base of a complicated hierarchy involving several levels with complex and divided mechanisms for linking across levels and between agencies. There are professional links from the very local level into the national system of medical organization, and of course into the Royal College of General Practitioners (RCGP) structure of education and training and development. There are few political links between the operational local service and the higher levels, other than through those professional linkages. Managerially the key linkages then flow from the district level to the locality, with weakly articulated political links between the district and the centre. Political directives are converted into managerial instructions, which confuses two sets of roles that may be better if kept more distinct. Both are distinct from the professional mechanisms, and fiercely resented when they have inevitable consequences for professional activity.

COMMUNITY HEALTH SERVICES

Until the early 1990s community health services were the responsibility of HAs but have been moved into community trusts since the reforms in the NHS. In both arrangements the traditional concept of organization assumes much more obvious relevance than was the case with general practice. In looking at these organizations it is important to remember that direct provision of primary care services forms only one part of the work of an organization with wider health care responsibilities. That breadth of concern also involves the organization in dealing with a much wider geographical area, and larger population, than the average general practice with its three or four partners and around 8000 patients. Given their range of functions and their scale and geographical spread community trusts organize their work through sections or divisions, often with specific professional responsibilities as the basis of organization, or a specific group of clients or patients as their focus. These divisions are in turn reinforced by geographical decentralization, usually into relatively small area-based teams to deliver services. This produces quite complex organizations and the implications of this are further amplified by the dominance of semi-professional work within the overall remit of the organization. Nursing functions form one dominant element, but residential and some domiciliary services require staffing by other, less highly trained people. The absence of a dominant professional group within the community trust, and the organizational mechanisms deemed essential to control a large, semi-professional and decentralized structure produce much more bureaucratic forms of organization. The public service ethos, given the absence of well established professional guarantees of performance, requires that the trust establishes alternative controls to manage performance and quality. These provide some security for clients, and equally importantly offer a basis for redress if problems do arise, but they can inhibit initiative, restrict activity and limit flexibility at the same time. The balance of these factors is complicated, but the successful operation of such organizations places a high premium on the quality of management, and on effective supervision. These in turn require high quality information systems and records, so that services that are complex and involve many staff provide managers and supervisors with the means to monitor activity, maintain standards and sustain reliability and accountability.

The fact that some groups of staff involved are seeking fuller professional status poses an obvious challenge to the dominant organizational pattern. The size of each professional group within the community trust is much greater than is the case in general practice, leading to a much stronger pattern of hierarchy within the organization with layers of management and supervision, which contrasts with the general practice model. This leads to a much clearer pattern of accountability within the organization and the need for clear systems to fulfil that accountability. Reporting looms larger and the machinery of control has to be clearer. Larger numbers of staff create a need for control over the quality and character of performance, which becomes an organizational issue as well as a professional one, with the criteria used to make such judgement sometimes being in conflict. This raises interesting issues in relation to control and accountability where work is undertaken in detached domiciliary or practice settings and where groups of staff are concerned to develop their professional status and autonomy.

Despite the creation of trust boards the concept of political direction at the local level seems not to be significant. Or, rather, it operates in a relatively opaque way, and its operation confirms the dominance of downward linkages from central government, which appoints members, rather than the two-way flow that characterizes local organizations based on formal democratic processes. The absence of effective linkages, certainly in terms of serious public influence on decisions, between the public and their community trust means that the mechanisms of accountability operate much more around staff relations with individual patients, and limit exchange to matters of particular cases rather than broader policy. The broader input into local policy making or strategic thinking is much more complex and restricted. This is profoundly involved with the power and influence patterns in the organization. Unlike general practice the nature of the relationships is influenced by the system of resourcing and the character of practice involved. In terms of resources and the control they involve, the new quasi-market means that the HAs and the GP fundholders for some services, are the source of funding for community services through the contract process, despite the latter also being a parallel provider. This system is of course still in its early days, and relationships are changing with growing experience of its operation. However, the external patterns of influence being created will involve trusts in key issues of quality control and standard setting and contract compliance, which will no doubt promote some reconsideration of their internal mechanisms already in place to deal with these issues. This is made more difficult by the detached, domiciliary nature of the work of many of those involved. Control over activity in the community is much more difficult than services based within and provided on fixed premises. In ideal typical terms it is a context that is suited to developed professional practice with the controls over practice arising from longer training, a clearer intellectual basis for action, and with the ethical and disciplinary controls asserted by the profession. In turn these are usually supported by complaints systems that allow particular issues to be dealt with if they do arise.

LOCAL GOVERNMENT SOCIAL SERVICES

Local authorities are different again. They are large scale organizations with a multiplicity of functions and an articulated system of local political direction and control. This political element is reflected in the resourcing system, which despite the dominant central contribution, and recent changes to limit local autonomy, does retain a tax raising capacity that gives decisions about spending a different significance for local politicians than is the case for their health care counterparts. The result is that the social work services that form part of extended primary care have to operate within the patterns of organization and control dictated by wider overall structure dominated by the big spending departments.

In terms of social services, the staffing, as with community nursing, is semi-professional in character, or in many cases non-professional, reflecting the diverse character of provision made within social services and reflected in the systems of control that are applied. There is strong internal accountability to the local authority driven ultimately by the political imperatives of local elections but in practice by the monthly committee round. This works at two levels. On the one hand it emphasizes the political direction of policy both at the broad level and at the intermediate level of decision usually left to management in many organizations. This gives politicians a much closer impact on service delivery. This is amplified at the detailed level by the fact that the representative process involves a more individualized contact around implementation where local councillors do act as conduits and advocates for constituents in relation to services, even those that are more highly professionalized.

Managerially speaking, these twin pressures require a more controlling structure within the local authority to fulfil the demands of accountability. This is formalized through the medium of the committee round and the formal council meetings where decisions are ratified and formalized. Of course a great deal is carried on outside that formal structure, but every service committee has a chair who plays a close role in the working of the department and social services are not an exception. The formal relationship gives the chair control over what happens within the service, but of course the informal processes make that a varying matter with roles in fact being reversed in some authorities while in others political control is paramount. Once again we need to keep the issue of implementation clearly in mind. Control and accountability, whether by managers or politicians, effectively depend on the quality of information against which to measure performance and compliance.

In professional services this is a complex issue. The nature of many aspects of complex interactive work that is the characteristic of some primary care is not easily susceptible to measurement, reportage or monitoring. Some aspects are and those are the ones that tend to form the basis of many systems of organizational control. These often run parallel to systems of professional super-vision designed to provide the input of professional support deemed essential in the early days of beginning practice, but con-tinuing throughout a career in the semi-professions where the prin-ciple of autonomy is less established. These twin systems are most apparent in the local authority setting, though they also apply in community health, and are only just appearing in the context of general practice.

IMPLICATIONS

These brief descriptions highlight a number of key features of organization that are significant when considering how several organizations can work effectively together to deliver an integrated care service, and operate more widely in developing future pro-vision and preventive strategies. The degree of professionalization is a clear concern, and interacts closely with the varying inter-vention of what might properly be called political processes. The different combinations produce quite distinct patterns of organiz-ation in each of the three cases, adding an extra dimension to the issue of interaction and involving a formal framework within which each contributor has to operate.

Management is the function that links those professional and political systems and its emphasis within the NHS reforms reflects a recognition of that role. The tension between those other roles presents a difficult challenge to managers, however, particularly where they assume a more apparent political role because the local politics are not formally established. This leads to different degrees of managerial autonomy in the three areas, which becomes signifi-cant when any medium or long term development is under review. Clear political direction can create opportunities for managerial initiative. Its absence can lead to conflict when the professionals perceive managers as acting politically, reflecting the absence of perceived political role-players locally, and a failure to understand the more politicized controls under which managers operate com-pared with professionals.

These problems surface most often in relation to discussion about the level and allocation of resources. They are made more difficult by the limitations placed on resource allocations, which are a fixed external factor at the local level. They are made still more difficult by the central government emphasis on the capacity for economies at the local level. This moves the debate from the difficult, but more comfortable area, of how to distribute additional resources to one where the issue is about what ceases to be done, or must be done very differently in order to save money for new activity.

The three key roles combine into three distinct patterns. The simplest model is of general practice where the professional has dominated by virtue of the substantial exclusion of both managerial and political actors who might impose constraints. Community nursing and social work offer more complex models in which all the roles are present but combined in quite different ways producing influence patterns that inhibit the freedom of action of all those involved.

CURRENT EFFORTS AT LINKAGES

This complex structure and the difficult linkages to which it gives rise has led to much effort going into schemes to try to achieve improvement without the basic structures being changed. These efforts have been reinforced by the recent reforms, which have introduced explicit attempts to make linkage a central feature of reform, largely through the mechanisms of the quasi-market that has been established.

The most obvious example is the effort being made to meet clear needs within the reformed system, despite the introduction of market mechanisms that theoretically should produce natural integration. One of these needs involves mechanisms for linking the centre with the locality for purposes of monitoring and control of the new system, and the other for securing aggregate local decisions that are sensitive to national targets and to wider local interests. These two roles are reflected in the HAs being given a responsibility for strategy, monitoring and support of local primary care activity. The roles are defined in ways that recognize the formal limitation of the power of the HA but also build on the capacity that arises from its control over some aspects of budgeting and resource allocation across primary and secondary care.

Other developments have been more particularly concerned with the purchasing role within the new system and facilitating the role of primary care within that new role. These involve the HA in a wide relationship with a range of agencies who represent the participants in what is here being called extended primary care. It is clear from the government exhortation on these developments that there is no single model being proposed and that different authorities are proceeding along different routes, though all with similar intention conditioned by the national rules. These models of locality purchasing relate specifically to the narrow function of primary care as the purchaser of secondary care, though interestingly they also cover the purchase of aspects of the wider primary care.

It is interesting to note that the basic functions of general medical service provision by GPs fall outside these locality schemes, though practices are being encouraged to include them within their plans for development. It is this provider element of general practice that poses the sharpest challenge for the new system as that forms the core of the independent system that has always prevailed but falls outside the new purchasing model. There is little evidence yet of efforts to impact on this area, but various areas of practice within the contract and *The Health of the Nation* strategy have been targeted and there is evidence about efforts to influence GP prescribing. In the case of the former there seems little doubt that adjusting the system of payment to reflect national priorities, and limiting those priorities to quantifiable activity of a basic kind, has produced results. Practice compliance is high, and there is evidence of speedy adjustment to rule changes in the area of health promotion activity within practices. The most recent proposals about primary care reform confirm government recognition of the need to begin to address this issue (Secretary of State 1996c).

Prescribing offers an alternative picture. Several efforts have been introduced ranging from the allocation of a formal prescribing budget in the case of fundholders, through indicative, but notional, prescribing targets for non-fundholders, to various incentive schemes to try to stimulate more efficient prescribing. Early evidence suggests that these different schemes have varied effects and that some have little effect at all (Walley *et al.* 1995). There is some evidence that prescribing among fundholders has been affected, at least in terms of the rise in levels of spending that has been contained (Wilson *et al.* 1996). In other respects the evidence shows limited response to initiatives and that their effect may perhaps be short-lived (Audit Commission 1996b).

CONCLUSIONS

If integration of provision and shared professional activity are the key hallmarks of future primary care, this discussion suggests that the current structures are likely to impose great restraint on development. The wide diversity of organization within the extended range of primary care makes joint work and shared responsibility more difficult than it need be. While this structure continues in place, reform of practice places a heavy burden on managers who play a key role in securing the interaction between agencies and between their professional staff. This role seems likely to develop even more in the future as Primary Health Care Teams emerge as a central vehicle for development. For social workers and community nurses this is at least consistent with their traditional ways of working, but for general practice it will clearly pose a sharp challenge to their autonomy and past working conventions. The same is true for the development of appropriate models of local political control, which are clear already in the social service field but non-existent in the context of general practice. Together these factors suggest a strong case for a more radical appraisal of how primary care is organized.

7

INTEGRATING EDUCATION FOR PRIMARY CARE

The systems of professional education for those involved in primary care have been developed to serve a health care system that is now changing rapidly, giving way to new ideas about primary care delivery and the wider role that it should play within the NHS. The existing systems have coped reasonably well with the demand for education and training during what with hindsight looks like a relatively stable period of service delivery and development. In the current more turbulent environment of changes in clinical practice, the NHS management structure, the internal market with or without fundholding, the organization and management of general practice and the character of a broader community-based primary care, they face more searching challenges. There is evidence of stress among professionals, recruitment difficulties in the case of general practice, and a widespread concern about the impact of change, which taken together suggest that the professions are not coping well with these challenges. Questions about the nature of the changes and the process of change of course arise. So too do questions about the capacity of current education and training to prepare professionals to meet the demands posed by the changes already in place, and by continuing change that seems likely during the remainder of this century and into the next.

INITIAL PROFESSIONAL EDUCATION

Professional education has not remained static over recent years. It too has experienced reform along with most other aspects of the NHS, but the extent and character of change has been limited by the general professional model that dominates education, though with important variations among the professions involved. In medical education, very belatedly given the history of changes in medicine and in the NHS, initial professional education is beginning to change in most university medical schools, directed centrally by the recommendations of the General Medical Council (GMC Education Committee, 1993). These change the emphasis of initial education to reduce the burden of factual learning and promote styles of learning, attitudes towards professional practice and relationships within that practice that reflect a recognition of much of the discussion in earlier chapters. In many medical schools this is being implemented by changing the balance of the approach taken in favour of problem-based and self-directed learning and involving much greater experience of community-based settings during training (Bligh and Parsell 1995). These developments seek to prepare tomorrow's doctors better for a lifetime of continuing learning and professional development. For those entering primary care, they reduce the emphasis on hospital practice and expose students to clinical situations and the community contexts in which they arise – both of which are fundamental to their future professional practice. It is too early as yet to be sure, but there is here the beginning of what should be a closer relationship between educational development and policy intentions for the development of the NHS.

In nursing, basic training has changed with Project 2000 (National Audit Office 1992) reflecting a clear adoption of the more traditional characteristics of professional education, with a move away from the heavy emphasis on extensive hospital based experience towards a more classroom based, intellectual approach, giving practical experience a more limited but more balanced role. This has no immediate direct relevance to primary care, but the greater emphasis on conceptual understanding, and on a wider range of subject matter, should develop deeper understanding that will help nurses coping with change, a capacity that is often less developed where experience has been the dominant mode of learning. If it also brings an enhanced sense of professional status then it may lead nurses to challenge the traditional pattern of medical dominance and could assist the introduction of a changed skill mix in the NHS generally and in primary care particularly. There are of course dangers in these changes. One is that conflict between the professions will follow from the assertion of extended roles by nurses, though changes in medical education and in the organization of care may limit that possibility. Another problem is the changes could lead to a deskilling of nurses in relation to their traditional tasks with a consequent need for other categories of nurse to provide those more basic practical services.

Social work has always involved a strong emphasis on classroom based education with more limited involvement in training placements to generate practical awareness and skills. More recently this balance has moved towards a larger component of practical experience. In part this is driven by questions of cost, but also reflects a wider government approach that favours the replacement of the intellectual basis of professional training with a much more experiential approach. This echoes very strongly the heavy emphasis on experiential learning within general practice, but of course in that case experience follows a very long period of basic education within medical schools that is not shared by social workers to the same degree. This has implications not only for the character of social work training, but also for the capacity to handle change. It is the analytic capacity derived from the more intellectual aspects of training that aids the adaptive process in professional roles, rather than mere experience, which by itself reinforces the commitment to current (and sometimes past) practice. In a climate where change and adaptation are required of staff, there is perhaps a need to reconsider the balance of academic and practical work within initial professional training.

Views about these changes are mixed, and their implications for the traditional areas of care for which the established training was seen as more appropriate will pose a clear challenge. Whatever the view taken, however, it is clear that the next generation of professionals in all areas of primary care will have come through a different initial experience than is the case with those already in practice, and they will be equipped in different ways for the changing roles they will face. One risk is that the length of professional training, and the pace of change in the NHS are such that these changes already in train are based on models of care, and patterns of working, that are changing again. Like much educational change in the past this reflects education reacting to the needs of current practice, and the constraints of its own limited capacity, rather than leading practice forward into new forms to meet anticipated future trends. The implications for continuing education are very evident.

CONTINUING PROFESSIONAL EDUCATION

Discussion in Chapter 5 showed clearly the nature of developing professional careers within primary care and the challenges they pose for the professions. New entrants in the future may have acquired more capacity for lifelong learning but the extent and character of some of the changes involved present severe challenges to those participating in continuing professional education and development. They will be central to future success, but are marginal to the current system of professional education.

There is increasing evidence that these extended career patterns are being recognized within general practice as posing challenges for continuing medical education (Irvine 1993). They also apply to the other primary care professions, most clearly perhaps in areas like management. This suggests that there are common professional issues that prompt consideration of generic models of professional development across primary care. They may even suggest a still more radical approach involving the idea of a new unified primary care profession where the common features dominate rather than the exclusive concerns of current earlier training. Such a change would recognize the increasing overlap in professional roles and the common themes raised around new knowledge, new ideas and the necessity for changed attitudes.

There are a range of skills, knowledge and attitudes that would be valuable to a primary care professional contemplating the kinds of career development involved but that are not readily available in the current system for continuing education. Some professionals have developed these wider skills through the necessity of undertaking more diverse activities, very visibly in the case of nurses and social workers who are promoted into formal supervisory and managerial positions, but no less significantly in general practice despite their less clear designation. Experiential learning is the dominant model of education applied in such cases, adapted from the traditional professional model, but not in these cases accompanied by the other coincidental educational processes that reinforce experience in the more traditional areas of work. At the extreme this approach reflects a view that there are no inherent skills and knowledge involved in these additional tasks that cannot be learned in this way. More moderately there is a tendency for professionals to claim that they already possess the appropriate skills and knowledge. Some of this reflects a narrow view of the tasks involved and one born of experience of them being undertaken badly, or having been less significant in the more stable traditional practice context. In large part, of course, these positions hide a simple defence of traditional professional autonomy which must assert that professionals can do it, because of the need to assert that others cannot do it to them. A corollary of such professional claims is the denial to other professions of validity in their claims for professional status, a position that has long inhibited interprofessional working within the more established core areas of primary care. It is important in addressing continuing professional development that the hard-won skills of other professions are recognized and used.

Basic to all of the extended roles involved in professional careers are communication skills. These are an interesting case in that they already form a core element of existing professional training in all these highly person-centred and case-based professions. This is most obviously the case in general practice where communication with the patient in the consultation forms a very substantial core of vocational training, and continues as a dominant theme in continuing professional education. It is significant in similar ways for social work and has become more so in hospital nursing where designated nurse responsibility for patients has increased its importance. The assumption is often made that the skills developed to deal with the patient/client contact are transferable into other contexts but clearly this is not a simple matter. While some part of the learning for the formal professional role is relevant in other settings, that relevance needs to be clearly understood and augmented. The key links, other than with patients, involve fellow professionals and other staff within primary care, professionals in secondary care and other related sectors, other agencies at a more managerial or bureaucratic level, the media, and the public at large. Communication in these wider contexts needs to be addressed directly, overtly taught and practised. In any profession heavily conditioned to experiential learning as the key to skill development, the transferability of skills and awareness from one situation to another should not be taken for granted. Neither should it be assumed that only the core primary care professionals understand these issues. There are clearly matters of agenda, language, style, timing and location that influence wider communication and that need to be understood. In many cases the key to communication lies in greater understanding of those being communicated with and the systems within which they have to work. This is often an area of great weakness among professionals whose own experience has been gathered exclusively within their own profession.

Equally central to the new NHS and to primary care are the core skills involved in research and development that lie behind the idea of an evidence-based practice, but also behind evidence-based development on a wider front. This is a complicated area, which, like communication, suffers from the fact that the research element of it is already seen to be integral to professional education. Initial education for all the primary care professions includes exposure to research and research findings, though the character and volume of the research and its value in terms of future practice varies widely. The opportunity to develop research skills and gain direct experience of doing research during professional training is, however, very limited, and for most entrants, the professional career emphasizes practice rather than research. In terms of the new primary care, this limitation is compounded by the fact that the dominant research model varies between the professions and there is limited mutual understanding and respect between the models. The medical research model, which also embraces nursing to a considerable degree, derives from secondary care and from the sciences setting a high premium on the idea of rigour and scientific method, which together limit the scope of research considerably. Social work on the other hand has its base in the more subjective arena of social science with its much greater tolerance of qualitative methodology and the development of grounded theory.

Research is particularly important in the context of primary care. Many of the features of the scientific canon are not easily applied in a context where diseases are less certain, where causes are more complex and where interventions cannot be isolated as they can in the context of much activity in secondary care. Clearly there are situations where such approaches can be used, but there are many more where the social sciences have much to offer both in relation to research methods and about relevant research questions. In terms of method qualitative research conducted without precise sampling frames and random selection of research subjects, subjective material handled in open ended ways, non-statistical material and indicative case analysis all form part of the spectrum of methods that might be used. For doctors and nurses, whose model of research respectability derives from medical school and teaching hospital experience, primary care is a difficult context for research. For all the professions, limitations of time and of opportunity compound the problems of limited background skill and capacity, and in any event many chose their career to avoid the demand that they should undertake research. In terms of research questions it seems clear from the discussion in Chapter 6 that issues about organization and management are just as important as those of professional practice, and involve their own research methods and styles.

This need not be a problem though it would create a difficult situation if the current emphasis on research and development were to promote the idea that all primary care professionals should be actively engaging in research. Some should be doing so, and the context for their research and how it can best be encouraged and developed are a challenge for primary care and for continuing education. There is a need to teach the research skills needed, and to encourage a climate in which research questions are shared and developed. This must be related to associated developments like reflective practice and medical audit, both of which share some related skills, and should naturally feed research agendas. Their extension into research depends on the wider cooperation of other professionals and other organizations and practices. That cooperation in turn depends on good quality recording and high quality information systems, both features that may need emphasis within the continuing education setting.

The issue of development is different. This is something in which all professionals should be engaged, as the application of best practice, and indeed best organization of that practice, is a central element in the provision of equitable and efficient care. Development does not involve research skills. It does, however, involve an understanding of the research process and methodology and a capacity in critical appraisal in order to evaluate research findings. It also involves a capacity to examine one's own current practice and its organization in ways that make it possible to relate research findings to the particular context and assess their relevance. It certainly demands a recognition that research and development are not essentially linked in terms of who undertakes them but by their close interrelation in practice. Development requires its own skills and appropriate attitudes, as well as adaptive organizations, to make it possible. Above all of course it requires research results to be adequately disseminated and accessible to the wider profession, a need that poses challenges to researchers and users alike. Meeting that need is another challenging aspect of the extended professional role.

Management skills are different again, though they do have a direct bearing on development. They seldom figure in initial professional training, not even as part of the information base for other learning. The good thing is that, like research skills, not all professionals need management skills. Where they do, it is helpful that adoption of a managerial role can be predicted and, in line with Houle's (1980) suggestion, planned and prepared for. The position is complicated in the context of wider primary care where

professionals do manage, but where professional managers analogous to those in the hospital sector are also employed. The issue
of a role for such professional managers is an important one and
the division of labour with professionals poses problems particularly where the latter see management and administration as iden-
tical activities. Whichever view is taken in that debate there will be
professionals who choose to take on managerial roles and for them
the educational issues are considerable. Such a decision comes close
to a change of profession rather than being a matter of professional
development and the challenge involved is consequently much
greater. This is recognized in the organization of nursing and social
work where becoming a manager involves ceasing professional
practice, but in general practice that would be seen by many as
undermining credibility and so inhibiting the ability to manage
other clinicians. The implications for lay managers are clear and
problematic, though such managers may be seen as less intrusive
than professionals managing as they do not bring their own models
of alternative professional practice to the table.

For those who do make the transition to management there is a
steep learning curve involved. The range of concerns of management, particularly in the smaller organizations that characterize
primary care, is extensive, partly because specialized management
is not justified by the scale of organization. Resource management
in its widest sense, embracing both the direct issues of finance, but
also involving the use of a widening array of human resources, is
one central concern. So too is the integration of the local concern
into the wider pattern of primary care at the broader level of the
health authority and of national policy. Questions of priority are
inherent in these tasks, but have assumed greater significance with
the reforms in the operation of the NHS. In short there is a range
of tasks that require skill in their application and that challenge professional autonomy directly. The necessary understanding of the
structure and dynamics of the decision making involved in organizations, and the special issues that arise within primary care, demand
considerable basic knowledge and analytic capability that have to
be developed late in professional careers.

For the many who do not make the transition to a management
role there remains a need to understand the concept of managed
activity. The fact that management requires systems of accountability and responsibility and involves planning and predictability,
is part of the learning of any professional intending to operate in
a managed setting. The traditional professional model has avoided

this, claiming full autonomy for the professional, and leaving a widespread attitude that professional activity is inhibited, rather than facilitated, by such management. A good reflection of this is the development of protocols to guide behaviour in practice, a development that may be pivotal to changing the way in which activity can be shared. Anecdotal evidence suggests that compliance with protocols poses problems even where professionals have shared in their design. The corollary of protocols of course is that professional behaviour should be modified to comply with them, and managerially, that compliance can be monitored in order to check on, and if necessary, adapt performance or protocol. Professionals need to understand what their managers can offer, and be able to work with them in combining managerial capacity and clinical direction in their work. This is complex as it does not involve learning to be a manager but rather to work within a managed system, which again raises the traditional questions of autonomy and clinical freedom and becomes a matter of attitude more than anything else. For a five partner practice with perhaps 20 employed staff, several attached and associated professionals, and between 10,000 and 12,000 patients this is a serious issue. Similar arguments could be mounted about financial management and about practice planning, both of which are specialized activities and both of which may pose limitations to the scope of professional autonomy.

Two other areas of skills were identified and linked in the earlier discussion of careers. One was the development of political skills relevant to many aspects of the extended role that might now be adopted by some primary care professionals. The other concerned the associated skills of advocacy, widely practised now though not always recognized as requiring the development of special skills. All the primary care professions operate as advocates, though it is much more common in general practice where the role of gatekeeper to other services leads naturally towards a form of advocacy. The character of the skills involved becomes obscured, however, as the activity is seen merely as referral and a part of extended case management. Where secondary care is the object of referral, competence is seen to spring from shared early learning in medicine and frequent interaction. Where other professions are involved the capacity for, and quality of, referrals confirms the need for more education and training. Fundholding, for those who have adopted it, has changed the .position somewhat by linking these issues to those of formal contracting for services and moving the debate from the traditional individual level to a more collective concern. This extends advocacy into the wider politics of health care, and may be central to the leading role of primary care in the new NHS.

One aspect of this wider role involves professional interests and this is widely institutionalized with a long history of successful advocacy, at least for the medical profession (Klein 1989). Where there is much less experience is in wider professional advocacy for patients and for the population as a whole. The activity that gave rise to many of the nineteenth-century reforms in health care and in health, discussed in Chapter 1, illustrates the importance of such advocacy in the less developed context of that time. Institutional development and professional specialization have moved the advocate role formally into public health, allowing other professionals largely to opt out of the process. This broken connection is unfortunate in that the basis for much advocacy is information, and that often lies in the knowledge gained in practice, which is not always adequately communicated to public health, and may lose impact when handled indirectly. This wider advocacy may be stimulated for general practice, and for other professions in primary care, by the commissioning process within the new purchaser/provider split. Contracting may be seen as an important opportunity for advocacy backed up by real power in terms of purchasing. This ties in with the earlier discussion about research and audit, and about information and communication, all of which are relevant to the effective exercise of advocacy. Needs assessment too becomes another essential skill if the debate is to be extended to deal with preventive activity and the needs of those not presenting to primary care as patients. The collective role of the Primary Health Care Team in such activity is obvious.

This discussion of skills may be readily extended into the knowledge required for successful engagement with the politics of a wider role for primary care in the NHS. Changes in the hierarchy of the NHS and independent status for many providers have created a need for knowledge both of institutions and of how they work. This applies both to NHS administration, community institutions and other professional bodies. The complex structures of the medical profession and of general practice are mirrored elsewhere, as we saw in Chapter 6, and interactive working demands close mutual knowledge of their detail. At this level there is also a need to be aware of what is happening in other areas, a need that sets a high premium on research, and of course on the effective management and dissemination of information.

One critical feature underlies all the issues discussed and that is the degree to which they apply to all the professions involved in primary care. The multidisciplinary character of primary care viewed from this perspective quickly gives way to the idea of an interdisciplinary perspective. At present this is made difficult by the very separate programmes of initial professional training for each of the professions, which reinforce division rather than promoting cooperation and shared activity. This makes multi- or interprofessional continuing education that much more difficult, though efforts are being made to move in that direction (Barr and Waterton 1996).

It will already be apparent that engagement with the skills and knowledge involved here is difficult. More difficult still, but essential to any radical change in practice and education, is change in attitudes on the part of the professions involved. Only broad general acceptance of the underlying principles of this approach will create a climate in which such skills and knowledge will be deemed relevant. Until the core roles and developing possibilities for each profession are clarified and accepted there is little hope for widespread change in education or in practice. Such acceptance, however, will not achieve change by itself. It may, however, stimulate response to the need for a wide ranging review of the continuing educational arrangements for primary care. Under the current system a GP wanting to extend his or her professional education in the ways discussed would find few structured opportunities to do so. For the nurses, social workers and managers involved the opportunities are even rarer in the absence of an equivalent at least to the PGEA system, which does give some focus to continuing education in general practice.

THE CURRENT SYSTEMS OF CONTINUING EDUCATION

These substantive needs have to be seen in relation to the current position with regard to continuing education in the three professions. There is much informal activity in all the professions focused around journal reading, informal discussion with colleagues and reflection on personal practice. This is an essential part of good professional development and needs to be fostered and improved, but is perhaps best suited to personal development and the more established core activities of traditional practice. The developmental aspects of a widening role within primary care demand more formal attention.

The importance of formal education is recognized in general practice, which already has a relatively elaborate system of continuing medical education, or what is increasingly being defined as continuing professional development. This system has important features that are in marked contrast to the other two professions. First is the existence of the Postgraduate Education Allowance (PGEA) paid since 1990 to those GPs who attend 30 hours of accredited education each year, with an added requirement that over a five year period they attend at least two courses concerned with health promotion, disease management and service management. This system ensures a reasonable level of formal involvement in continuing education, but detailed studies of the system indicate very diverse patterns in the provision made for GPs both in terms of style, content and quality. The system is administered, not provided by, the Regional Advisers in General Practice who accredit and approve courses being offered. Uncertainty about the quality of the system has more recently led to the appointment of locally based GP tutors whose task is to manage the system, and who, as their role becomes established, are seeking better to meet emergent needs and to promote ideas about how continuing education is best undertaken.

Nursing and social work have no such system in place, nor are resources provided in this earmarked way, which is perhaps a further sign of the relative position of general practice, and of course the different formal employment structure that it enjoys. The result is a much more uncertain process within these other professions. Courses are offered which deal with parts of the agenda discussed and also with the continuing core needs of any professional activity. There is a much less localized focus for much of this activity, which of course militates against the continuing informal contact among professionals, and which reinforces continuing education in the best examples. The absence of earmarked financial support explains some of that difference, with nurses and social workers suffering from the varied capacities of health authorities, trusts and local authorities to support attendance and thereby promote continuing education. Where education conflicts with service in the demand for resources it is easy to underestimate the value of education.

It is argued here that these systems are not an adequate basis for developing the capacity to cope with the emergent primary care-led NHS. Certainly there would be wide agreement that it is not simply a matter of extending the PGEA system from general practice to the other professions, even if that could be resourced currently, which is almost certainly not the case. That might help the demand side of the educational equation in that it could provide a basis for nurses and social workers to pay for courses and other educational opportunities. But demand is not the problem. Most professionals recognize their continuing needs, both to update and to develop and extend their capacities. The problem lies in the service demands that inhibit them from taking time out to do so, but equally important the absence of an effective supply side in continuing education to cater for their widening professional needs.

THE FUTURE

The implication of this discussion is a need to consider the future of professional education in a way that reflects understanding of the character of that education, but that also reflects the realities of the new primary care. It must take on board the breadth of competence involved in primary care, and the complex interdisciplinary character of that care.

The new approach to primary care calls for professionals equipped to engage with changing and widening roles and relationships. These, as has been shown, involve more interdisciplinary work, a general engagement with new disciplines, and a more selective, in-depth opportunity for some professional staff to engage with aspects of the widening agenda. This requires professional education to recognize the shared concerns involved in basic professional practice, but also the blurred boundaries around professional roles as careers develop and a more elaborate model of primary care comes into play. Educational needs assessment in such a context forms a central part of any developed continuing education. Professionals may be able to assess their own needs in their traditional areas of work where they have a good initial grounding and accumulated further experience. Where new activities are involved, and they have little background knowledge, they will need closer guidance in the task. Who does what in the wider context of the emerging primary care becomes an open question, and the answer may vary over time, or with the particular context. In such a situation the role of teacher/facilitator assumes much greater significance.

One radical approach to this situation would be the development of a new profession for primary care, bringing the current professions together but equipping them to fulfil the basic generic roles involved. This would recognize common elements within their separate systems of current training and would respond to the fact that much training, especially in medicine, is remote from the subsequent needs of primary care practice. It would, of course, resolve the interdisciplinary difficulties in the current system although care might be needed to avoid transforming such arguments into intradisciplinary problems for the new profession. Such a system might provide a more appropriate set of primary care generalists who could meet many current needs. Their level of skill, and of training, would leave areas of more specialized need to be filled in other ways. Referral for specialist attention within primary care might become normal and would require some professionals to develop skills to a higher level. Management and supervision would also be required and the hierarchy involved would demand further training for those who were to exercise such roles. This would reflect the range of career progressions within existing primary care discussed in Chapter 5, but would provide a more coherent and cost effective basis for their development. It would secure greater congruence between education and training and the main focus of professional activity. It would also assist the development of more appropriate preparation for the tasks that are currently undertaken without such preparation. It would require dramatic changes in the existing training and education provision.

Even without such radical change, current professional education and training must be transformed. If a single profession is not to emerge, the current professions at least need to develop a much higher capacity for working together. Initial professional training is likely to be more difficult to change in this direction but some conscious effort needs to be addressed to provide common elements to all those involved. Modular programmes in education and training are now more common and more readily allow for such development. The advent of more community based learning could provide a basis for some shared opportunities during those periods. It will be ironic if the new curricula in medical schools involve medical students being taught by other professions within the community, but not alongside students preparing for careers in those professions. If such developments were possible they would greatly ease the path to multi- or interprofessional learning in continuing education. If they are not, continuing education will have to build on the current diffused efforts being made to cater for joint learning (Barr and Waterton 1996).

If this is to happen more widely it almost certainly needs the professions to move closer in the way in which their continuing education is organized. Current continuing education militates against this. Provision is episodic in character, short sessions or courses predominate, and in general practice the system of funding emphasizes individual interests and voluntarism in directing uptake. In the other professions some of the same factors apply, but the dependence for funding on employer support often dictates that the topics favoured will reflect employer or organizational needs rather than those of professional staff, especially if those involve more radical agendas. Whichever system is involved the overriding problem is the unpredictability, both of uptake and of what is taken up. This makes overall planning difficult. The higher degree becomes the main route to organized continuity of learning, but is very expensive both financially and in terms of time commitment. Individual portfolio based learning goes some way towards meeting the need for continuity, but the supply side of current continuing education makes the planning of a portfolio very difficult.

The significance of this lack of capacity for systematic planning and coherent development is that it flies in the face of Houle's (1980) principle that professionals need organized educational opportunities to prepare for key career transitions. All the professions cater for this need in relation to the adoption of formal teaching roles within initial professional training, and for some aspects of professional practice, but it is remarkably absent from the more diverse developmental needs of professional practice. Planning, both for employing organizations and individual professionals, depends on a predictable provision of educational opportunity so that the constraints on uptake can be overcome.

The connection between education and practice involved in such forward planning also applies to the wider interaction around development issues. Interdisciplinary education without the reinforcement of interdisciplinary practice is likely to limit the quality of learning, especially where educational inputs are modest in scale. The reverse is also true in that the learning process is greatly enhanced where professionals bring experience of interdisciplinary practice into the classroom. This calls for changes in the structure of primary care itself; these are dealt with in Chapter 8. It also calls for education that is sensitive to the realities of practice. Education can lead practice, but where practice lags behind, education may need to address issues in new ways that recognize the need for more basic understanding of principles and that cater for the need for organizational change rather than implementation in unchanging organizations. This is not a call for education simply to reflect practice, but for education to be aware of where practice is, and what is needed to move that practice forward. Practice-based education is one approach to this problem, and is currently receiving much support within general practice. The scope of such development in relation to the future of primary care may be more limited in the sense that innovatory practice is not widespread, and more importantly, that diffusion of ideas widely throughout primary care is not easily reconciled with this model.

The alternative approach is for education and training to become a more specialized activity and to become evidence-based in exactly the same way as is expected of practice. This will be difficult to achieve in a primary care system where research is currently limited, where the pace of change is rapid, and where one early aim for future continuing education is to develop the necessary research and development skills. The challenge is twofold. On the one hand, professional education, especially continuing education, must reflect the cutting edge of best practice in both traditional terms and in relation to innovatory practice. This will involve good, innovatory practices in an even wider range of activities than at present as they become the object of research and possibly of educational attachments for established professionals. It will also involve efforts to link existing research in other fields, like organization and management or community development, with parallel development within primary care. This is made easier by the fact that primary care differs in its particular features but shares many common elements with other activity. Small organizations do have features in common and so too do organizations concerned with responsive and accountable relationships with the public. Awareness of these parallels is one key stage in the development of a similar awareness across the range of primary care activity.

Development must also involve best practice in education, which demands parallel expertise drawing on its own professional research base. If education is to offer appropriate insights into better educational practice and innovatory organization, someone needs to be researching those examples, and that research must feed back into the process of educating professionals. The current tendency to borrow concepts from general adult education is highly desirable, but needs associated research activity to underpin their effective translation into the professional context. Professional needs must be served by education and not bent to meet the demands of any particular model of education.

Two further features are necessary. One is the need for the system to become much more a national one rather than a loose coming together of diverse local practice. The goals of equity and optimal care demand a greater uniformity of practice, and a system where innovation will be diffused widely when it is demonstrated to be desirable. Much of the current variation in practice arises from the failure to legislate for some changes and to leave them to individual adoption, and the more general acceptance of the concept of education being controlled by the professions, particularly in medicine. While the latter may be desirable, the demands of equity and of cost-effectiveness may begin to dictate another agenda that will clash with that principle. Professional control may be maintained, but the professions will need to grapple with these issues and engage more openly with questions of content, participation and accreditation. The principles currently being applied in initial professional training in these respects will need to be applied across the professions and in their continuing education.

The structure that best suits these needs is not currently in place, but initial education and training does offer a base on which to build. The universities currently house the diverse elements that are needed to develop such an approach, and the model of linked practice, research and teaching is well established. It is currently under-developed in the area of continuing professional education in primary care. University departments do provide courses and more structured programmes within continuing education for the professions, and general practice has an administrative system associated with postgraduate medicine. At present the system reflects practice in failing to make the connections across disciplines and between levels. Many of the criticisms applied to primary care could also be applied to the universities. However, the opportunity is there to reshape university organization to reflect models of integrated primary care practice much more easily than in the community setting where heavy service demands have to be met. Schools of primary care, or of community service, could link disciplines at several levels. Their research would be influenced by such connections, their teaching would be more easily organized around interdisciplinary concerns and the model for professional practitioners would fit the needs of future practice much more precisely than do current arrangements.

Such changes will not be made without resources being made available any more than they will be within primary care itself. Organizational change is costly, at least in the short term when transition costs arise. In the long term it seems likely to deliver savings as boundaries blur and flexibility becomes more normal. If one looks at the current resources spent on continuing education they would provide some capacity to facilitate this transition if they could be spent differently. If they cannot the danger is that education and training will imitate practice in enjoying some random innovation, but not the coherent development called for in a primary care-led NHS.

8

A NEW ORGANIZATION FOR PRIMARY CARE

The discussion so far has indicated several features of the historic organization of the NHS and of primary care that in part account for the failure of past reforms. It is argued here that unless those features are addressed then the Conservative government's reforms will fall well short of the goals outlined by Starfield (1992), goals that are evident in the continuing rhetoric about the primary care-led NHS. This is important because these considerations bear directly not only on the issues of quality and equity, but also on those of efficiency and effectiveness, which now loom larger in the debate about primary care. They are made more significant by the probability that the changing demands of the volatile environment for primary care seem likely to impose a continuing need for adaptation and development.

The earlier analysis suggests five important, and interrelated, aspects of the current system that need to be taken into account in any restructuring:

1 the fragmentation of the system, between levels and between sectors and professions at all levels;
2 the profusion, and perhaps confusion, of roles within primary care and the varied power and influence of the key professional role players within the different subsystems of care;
3 the difficulty of efficient and effective resource allocation in a primary care system in which central allocations are divided between departments of state, and where consequent related local spending depends on different organizations and methods and styles of budgeting;
4 the inadequate linkage between policy and implementation in this complex system, both in terms of the connecting mechanisms,

the information flows and the unforeseen consequences this can have for patients;

5 the varied levels of spatial concern within primary care, leading to care that concentrates on individual cases or very small population groups, while planning and resource allocations struggle with area-wide concerns, losing important links between primary care delivery and public health planning.

Of course these are not new problems. They have been present within the NHS and the different sectors of primary care for many years, inhibiting the impact of reform over a long period. Efforts have been made to overcome them at various levels. At the macro level they have involved policy decisions about priorities and about budget allocations, but those most closely involved in using the resources have exerted their influence to protect existing interests and prevent what would have been more radical solutions if they had been implemented more effectively. At the micro level some progress has been made, usually led by innovative individuals concerned with improving services and usually having to operate in spite of, rather than because of, the system. Examples of innovative practice and improved professional relationships within primary care are to be found, and they illustrate very clearly the significance of the five principles listed above. They also serve to illustrate how difficult it is to diffuse such ideas throughout the present system and how much the structures militate against widespread adoption of new practices. This pattern of change, and the limitations on adoption, has been confirmed by the evidence drawn from the Conservative government's reforms. They have led to new ways of working, and evidence of desirable changes being made among fundholders in the general context of purchasing secondary care, and in the new community care arrangements. They have also demonstrated the limitations of the reform process in extending such practices more widely.

In the last chapter it was argued that one step towards a more radical advance in primary care would involve changes in professional education to prepare various groups for their role in a reformed service. The systems model and the connections it highlights suggest that education by itself will not be sufficient to secure radical reform. The changing knowledge base, skills and attitudes of primary care professionals will need new structures within which to practice, if they are to be reinforced by experience and have the beneficial effects intended in a primary care-led NHS.

INNOVATION IN PRACTICE

In the absence of any thoroughgoing reform of the existing structures of primary care, some of those involved have rightly opted for the pragmatic expedient of seeking new ways of working within the current constraints. A number of examples now exist that demonstrate the scope of what is possible within primary care even with its present organization. At the same time such efforts confirm the limits of this model of change and the significance of the issues highlighted above.

Fundholding provides a good example. The scheme was voluntary, and initially limited to larger practices, both factors that might have been expected to recruit more innovative doctors who shared the view that the traditional patterns and relationships in primary care needed to change. They might have been expected to share the aims of a scheme that was explicitly designed to change the relationship between primary and secondary care, a central plank of a primary care-led NHS. Though less explicit at the outset, they might also have accepted the opportunity provided to pursue the possibility of fundholders working more effectively with community nursing and other related professional services. Aspects of the scheme, particularly control of the prescribing budget, were also expected to change patterns of prescribing with possible consequences for the conduct of practice itself.

Evidence from practice among fundholders confirms these possibilities, but suggests that although the scheme has produced innovation, such changes have not been widely diffused. The variety of performance and approach among fundholding practices is in some ways the most striking feature of that reform so far, echoing very clearly the character of the previous system with its emphasis on practice autonomy and consequent tolerance of diverse practice. Within the varied pattern of change the evidence suggests that there is more compliance with changes around those areas of the management of care that have been built into the government guidelines and the *Patient's Charter* (Department of Health 1995b). Appointment systems and waiting times have been improved along with some other features of referred care, but much appears not to have changed significantly. The widely adopted changes reflect a response to direct government initiatives, and sometimes to financial incentives, as much as to the budgetary freedom and responsibility inherent in the concept of fundholding. This may reflect the significance of a new breed of high quality managers brought into general practice by the advent of fundholding. They seem often to have been the instrument of change, and sometimes the catalyst, rather than the fundholding GPs playing that role, a pattern that would tend to limit changes in directly clinical matters (Audit Commission 1996). This should not detract from the gains that have been made and the innovations that have occurred in some practices and are being continued in the total purchasing pilot schemes (Henry and Pickersgill 1995).

One explanation for the limited gains may be that fundholding has been one of the more divisive reforms in terms of the professional response to its introduction. Polarization of opinion among GPs about fundholding, and the very public critique that it creates a two-tier service, may well have limited more radical adoption of some changes despite the evidence that primary care has always been multitiered in its quality. One consequence of divided opinion has certainly been a search for alternative forms of organization through which to involve GPs in the purchasing role that is central to the new NHS market and the pivotal role of primary care within it. This has led to a number of developments, multifunds being one that brings together several practices, giving a collective relevance to purchasing decisions that cannot be obtained through a single practice. Another is the various consortium arrangements established to provide GPs with an opportunity to become involved in health authority purchasing decisions.

Each of these developments is interesting in reflecting some of the needs that are evident in the reformed NHS. They provide a basis for feeding primary care awareness of health care needs into decisions about wider populations and limiting some of the risks of multitier provision continuing as a result of the varying competence among a large number of purchasers. The health authority (HA) operates at the right geographical level to reflect the need and take the opportunity to seek greater equity, and these arrangements add the key ingredient of information about health need that arises from the GPs' clear awareness of their patients' needs. This input of information lies at the heart of the reform process, as without it, decisions to meet demand, and their consequences for provision in other sectors, will not reflect the realities of local need as it is experienced on the ground. The issue remains as to whether these systems cater adequately for the transfer of that local knowledge into a sensitive purchasing system, or whether they merely provide notional capacity at the point of contract, and have little impact on the management of the process of delivering care. The problem with this model is that the consortia come together for the limited purpose of purchasing. While the contracting process between primary and secondary care is important, it deals in broad aggregate terms, leaving detailed clinical practice to continue as the more significant factor in determining actual patterns of care. This is particularly the case where changes in primary care are called for as a result of the changed interface with secondary care. Unless the consortia develop a capacity for collective response to such needs, then the benefits of collective purchasing will not flow back into general adjustments in primary care.

Community care is another area in which significant changes have occurred in joint working since 1990. The arrangements for planning care mean that local social services and other agencies in primary care have to work together and engage with secondary care around the discharge of patients. This has produced new contacts and new relationships and has extended the scope of mutual awareness across extended patterns of care. Of course, as with all reforms, experience has been varied, and resource constraints and local factors have limited the extension of provision and the wide adoption of best practice (Lloyd *et al.* 1995). Resource constraints would promote difficulties in any structure of provision, but its effects are amplified by the divisions of labour and resource contribution involved in such diverse agencies. Once again reform illustrates what managerial and professional collaboration can achieve, but how present structures make cooperation difficult.

Different from fundholding and community care, which have been driven by an explicit political agenda, and have been the subject of considerable debate, there are other developments that reflect a more conventional model of change. These form part of a normal process of development, though at the time of writing many seem to be driven by the need to respond to significant changes within secondary care that have been triggered by the reforms. They also depend in some cases on the chance availability of capital funds to refurbish old or to build new facilities. This reflects a long-standing feature of the public sector where much reform is driven by the opportunity to develop capital projects, with continuing revenue costs always a problem in the longer term. Despite the limits of such opportunities the take up of development reflects the clear wish on the part of some professional participants to develop shared capacity within primary care. Developments certainly raise the level of mutual awareness among the professions and the agencies involved, changing patterns of service delivery as a result, and moving some secondary care services into community settings. Coincidentally such developments can change the pattern of patient use of primary care and can provide extended access in areas where conventional services are not readily engaged by difficult populations. These are all desirable goals and are one response to the fragmented character of current primary care discussed earlier.

A report on two such developments, one a physical resource centre, and the other a resource network without any formal building as its focus, reflects the difficulties of development and the features essential to success (Gordon and Hadley 1996). In the main it seems to be the community services and nursing who are leading the way in these developments and because of that they are often managerially rather than professionally led. The obstacle to development of this kind is reported to be the difficulty of convincing GPs of the desirability of such resource centres. Once the centre is established it seems that those GPs involved, however reluctantly in the initial stages, do develop new ways of working, both with one another, and with other services involved. The dynamics of development, however, indicate how difficult the process is, and how expensive it would be to replicate as a general model for change.

Part of the explanation may lie in the fact that these developments took place and were stimulated by the fact that existing primary care services in the areas concerned were not very good. This may account in part for the difficulties that arose from the fact that 'the GPs were all relatively new to the idea of teamwork, were developing their understanding of the primary health care team, and not all of them had regular practice meetings' (Gordon and Hadley 1996: 59). In the case study reported this was compounded by the lack of knowledge among the GPs about community services, reflecting on their exercise of their traditional gatekeeper role that should depend crucially on such knowledge. Ultimately the authors conclude that 'GPs will only do what they want to do' and their contractual status clearly reinforces that attitude. It seems that 'committed, clever and patient community services staff' can effect change by gradual and subtle influence (Gordon and Hadley 1996). Such a model is, however, unlikely to diffuse easily throughout primary care. It seems that current attitudes require that each case must develop its own particular rationale if it is to be accepted. The approach seems somewhat inconsistent with the current vogue for evidence-based practice though entirely at one with the history of innovation.

Polyclinics are a particular version of the resource centre, bringing together a variety of providers, conventionally under one roof. They are currently under discussion in many areas, and are particularly significant in areas where secondary care resources are being reduced, as in London and other inner cities. These are coincidentally often areas where primary care has not historically developed very far and where patients have relied on the accident and emergency (A and E) departments of hospitals as an alternative to primary care. As with the general model of resource centres they tend to reflect a capital spending, building-led approach to solving the problem, and the variety of models adopted perhaps reaffirms the limitations of the model in changing attitudes and practice. The tolerance of variation of course allows professionals to participate without undue threat, and the experience of being involved may change practice over time, but the key features that seem essential to their operation confirm the difficulty of that transition.

An example in Westminster illustrates the gains that can be achieved, but also the key requirements that have to be met to achieve success. Shared services, good access for patients, clear growth of knowledge on the part of professionals involved and ready adjustment by patients to the new arrangements all suggest the value of the model. Management of the development process and of the polyclinic, once established, are the central needs however, even assuming the necessary 'sharing of the vision' by all those involved. Development demands strong management to 'keep everyone involved and feeling committed' and after that phase to 'continually review activities, to build on knowledge all the time, and not be afraid of changing and remodelling services as the need arises' (Gordon and Hadley 1996: 78).

Another area of related development lies in the area of teamwork within current general practice. Changes in general practice have extended the range of staff involved, both employed within practices and attached from other agencies. The potential for teamwork inherent in these developments has been heavily reinforced by the very positive support of the RCGP for the Primary Health Care Team as the way forward. As with most other aspects of primary care the resulting pattern of changing practice is varied. There are clearly some effective teams in operation and changes in working practices follow their development. There are more cases where the constituent members of an extended team are in place but where interdisciplinary working is much slower to develop. As always there are others for whom the concept of team would be difficult to use in relation to their operation.

This uneven development reflects the same inhibitions that apply to the more detached development of resource centres. All the issues of organization discussed in Chapter 6 conspire to make teamwork difficult and they are reinforced heavily by the current organization and character of professional education and training. Chapter 7 suggested ways in which this latter difficulty might be addressed but attention also needs to be given to alternative organization for cooperation.

AN INTEGRATED FUTURE

Most of these changes reflect attempts to overcome the fragmentation and the barriers that inhibit the interprofessional development of current primary care delivery. They display very clearly the significance of the boundaries built into the current system of primary care and the dynamics of two processes involved in dealing with them. Where interagency development is involved, the problems are clear, and it seems in many cases that reform is being led by those within community health or local social services rather than from within general practice. In such cases the process involves considerable effort to persuade GPs to become involved, usually it should be said, with positive results once they have been persuaded. The evidence seems to confirm that once joint working is established, then everyone recognizes its value and begins to change their own practices to accommodate the new opportunities. Where development emerges within general practice, both the advantages gained and the difficulties experienced are less visible because of the setting. They do still exist, however, and reform seems to depend on the leadership of an innovatory GP, or in some cases a group of partners. This model of reform seems to be accepted as the appropriate and inevitable model of development for general practice, despite its limitations when primary care is taken as a whole.

Given both the historical and more recent experience, neither model of process suggests easy dissemination or early adoption of the changes by others within primary care. Evidence based organizational change does not seem to be the prevailing norm, and indeed there is some suggestion that development is seen to depend on emphasizing the particular characteristics of local circumstances rather than the universal issues involved. This reinforces the tradition that asserts the uniqueness of practice rather than the common characteristics that run across primary care. The ability to develop a programme of more general reform is weakened by this attitude and yet the wider picture suggests a clear need for more generic change. In the circumstances it seems useful to consider the lessons of current experiments and to ask whether there are more general changes that would better engage the barriers to change and facilitate quicker diffusion of ideas and more widespread adoption of changes that have proved worthwhile.

The key to such changes seems to lie in three factors. One is the significance of organizational boundaries and their constraints on current professional roles, reinforcing opposition to change when it is suggested. Another is the associated separation of budgets to coincide with boundaries leading to arguments about who is responsible for paying for services and causing responsibility to be defined by resource constraints rather than best use of combined resources. A third is the complex geography of primary care and the fragmentation that inhibits bringing together the detailed concerns of practice patients with those of other practices or agencies and with wider populations.

The continuing relevance of all these factors arises from the historical failure to address primary care as a singular focus and to tackle the difficult political questions involved in applying that focus. The discussion suggests that there is a clear case for a single authority to be responsible for primary care rather than to continue with the present system of fragmented responsibility. Moves in this direction have, of course, been suggested on several occasions in the past. The Royal Commission in 1979 expressed itself in favour of developments that would lead to the 'concentration of catchment areas and movement towards zoning or sectorisation' and towards 'planning and delivery of coordinated patient care by hospital and community services for a given population in a given locality' (Merrison 1979: para. 7.5). They stopped short of recommending a single authority for primary care, but hoped that boundaries would blur in the process of development, leading to much more integrated practice; of course this has happened to some degree in the situations discussed earlier. The RCGP has also expressed itself in favour of a primary care authority (Waine 1992). It envisages the development of an authority to oversee primary care, but does not see the need for changes in the structure of general practice or of the other services involved, merely that all staff contracts would be held by the new authority. While this would create greater coherence at the subsystem level it leaves open the question of how compliance with that strategy is secured at the level of practice. If GPs continue as self-employed while other staff become primary care authority employees this seems unlikely to resolve the difficulties currently experienced.

Such support for reorganization, and the evidence about conventional practice, suggest that the time may have come to grasp the bull by the horns and seek a fully integrated model of care, catering for the horizontal links necessary at all levels, but also the links between levels that are so fundamental to future success. Historically the argument for such development has ground to a halt on the basis that there is no agreement among the established participant interests about where such a unitary organization should be located within the overall system of public service. Or, more accurately, there has been no agreement to recurrent suggestions that local government would provide a suitable home for such development. The analysis given above offers some guidance about location and seeks to avoid special pleading for any of the pre-existing structures that have in any case failed to deliver the level and quality of integrated care which are desirable. This allows us to isolate those features of organization which are important in any reform, although it may be that the features interrelate in ways that make optimal solutions difficult to achieve.

First and foremost is almost certainly the need to find a system that will overcome the interprofessional rivalries and conflicts that have marked past primary care, and to inhibit the dominance of any single profession, certainly in terms of traditional professional roles. The suggestions made about professional education would of course take us a long way in this direction. The idea of a new professional role as primary care specialist with several levels of skill development facilitating a competent multifaceted service delivery, and the availability of sensitive specialist advice from more highly trained and experienced practitioners, would take us even further.

In the absence of such a radical change there are a number of factors that need to be incorporated in any new structure. There is a need for organization at the strategic level of the primary care subsystem where key decisions are taken about priorities and about the allocation of resources to service them. This is where the budgetary issues among the contributory services can be handled with some capacity to adjust allocations between areas of work that have different but interrelated needs. It is also the level at which the number and location of professional staff, and decisions about the appropriate mix of skills, can be addressed in a coherent and organized way rather than relying on the coincidence of local interests leading to more optimal allocation. This strategic role would be greatly facilitated by a single authority with a wide geographical remit to provide, rather than purchase, primary care. The scale would depend on the pattern of the national allocation of resources and the nature of the area involved, but local government experience suggests that the county council structure, both non-metropolitan and metropolitan, would best fit the bill. Even before their abolition in 1986 the large metropolitan counties did not have these functions, but that was because service delivery was the focus rather than strategic resource allocation, and small scale was seen as essential to the former.

Decision making on that scale to meet those high level strategic needs would require careful organization of the service delivery aspects of primary care. Discussion so far has emphasized the importance of implementation of policy and suggested that, given other developments, linking both within a single organization may be the logical way forward. This would assist some of the necessary aspects of future primary care. Each organization would be big enough to accommodate the necessary range of different professional skills, but also to maintain a critical mass of specialists in each profession within the organization. This would facilitate personal development and, more especially, continuing professional development, both of which depend crucially on peer contact being available within the organization. This is the context within which professional issues arise and where shared reflective practice exposes learning needs but also provides opportunities for them to be met. The large organization involved at this level would involve a large population that would accommodate the staff–client ratios necessary in some of the more marginal services within primary care.

This highlights issues about service delivery and the qualities inherent in the current structure of practice. The great virtue of the current system of general practice is its accessibility to those who need to use it, and this accessibility must be maintained in the new structure. This need not involve independent organization of services however, given that the changes are intended to tackle the difficulties raised by the boundaries drawn around independent organizations. Devolved service delivery could be built into the system, as it is already in some areas of primary care. These current arrangements help, but do not guarantee close working relationships, but the creation of multidisciplinary teams within the one primary care organization would facilitate both contact and accessibility. The character of the area is an important aspect of this development, however, and the simple device of bringing two or three general practices together may not provide the appropriate answer. The scale will be one determinant of provision but so too will be its socio-economic character. Large areas would mean more heterogeneous populations, which would involve a more balanced pattern of need and demand, which would bring advantages in terms of overall resources, allowing for local decision to provide sensitive guidance about detailed allocation. The resource centre model reflects this structure but does not usually involve merging of identity and accountability among those involved.

An added advantage of the less fragmented structure would be the enhanced ability to deal with an area as a whole, avoiding the overlaps and confusions in the current system. This would be further enhanced if the area boundaries could coincide with some sense of community involving other shared features in terms of social, economic and public service concerns. The holistic view involved in the 'patch approach', echoing the wider shared concerns at the more strategic level, would enhance other possibilities. Significant issues related to common population needs, and the wider public health questions, which involve services other than primary care, would be better addressed in such a context. It would help to forge connections that were strong in the nineteenth century but have been lost since then.

Such a devolved system of patch and team based primary care will need to guard against the heavily bureaucratic controls that mark the current system in all of its forms. The heavy direct interventions of nursing and social work, and the many indirect controls emerging in general practice can inhibit professional work and innovatory practice. The scale and character of the proposed structure could avoid such features. The strategic level would be large enough to involve professional inputs to policy making and the development of shared guidelines for best practice. It would also be large enough to employ high quality managers with the sensitivity and skills to engage the dialogue with professionals about the proper balance between autonomy and accountability that must be the hallmark of public sector organization. This would be replicated at the level of service delivery where the multiprofessional character of the teams, and the closer relationship that they could have with non-professional staff working within the same patch, could allow for looser systems of formal control. Budgetary limitations would be necessary, and quality controls would need to be put in place, but a good deal of autonomy should be possible in day to day practice. In any case the significance of the change may not be as great as some professionals fear. Nurses and social work staff already exercise a good deal of effective autonomy within a highly structured system of apparent control. Examination of general practice suggests that limits on autonomy are currently more real than the rhetoric suggests, and that the substance of practice has survived many of the recent changes so that organizational change might not be as intrusive as it would seem.

The corollary of such change, if it were to be introduced, would be the need to organize carefully to manage the interface between managerial and professional interests, and the political context in which they are played out. This will be a more complex task than at present and will clearly pose a considerable managerial challenge. It will be helped by changes in professional education and by the extended possibility of some professionals moving into full time managerial roles. It will also involve recognition of the need to recruit, train and develop a cadre of managers with the skills and awareness to manage complex professional activity sensitively. The dialogue between managers and professions would require a good deal of mutual sensitivity but the messages emerging from practice both in terms of fundholding and other developments in shared primary care show that this can happen. The filling of these management posts would be a significant task, and they would not necessarily be found among the current staff within the NHS or local government. One difficulty of the reforms since 1980 has been the emphasis on management, coupled with the notion that the existing management, brought up in a quite different NHS environment, would be appropriate to the new task. Given the emphases of the old system this was inherently unlikely, and simple recruitment of managers from business, where sensitive management of professional staff is not in any case usual, does not provide an easy answer. This is now being compounded by attempts to reduce the cost of NHS management rather than recognize the need for quality in this most vital role within the new primary care-led service.

Overcoming the obvious hurdle of manageability in the new system would be aided greatly by a reorganization that recognized the legitimacy of political decisions in health care, both nationally and locally. At the time of writing, the absence of an effective local politics in health care leaves the way open for national politicians to dictate broad policy and in many cases much more detailed local priorities. This is perfectly proper and legitimate, though it may be thought undesirable by some. When the debate moves to implementation at the local level the absence of clearly formalized local politics means that managers are often left to fill essentially political roles. This is reflected in the appointment of many trust directors and health authority members who see themselves playing managerial rather than political roles. This division of labour needs to be clarified if managers are to avoid being seen as the instrument of political will, rather than as the interpreters of that will into effective clinical and associated practice. Essentially managers and professionals work together to make best use of limited resources within established political guidelines about priority. If politics is imposing inappropriate constraints on professional action, it is for managers and professionals together to say so and clarify that the implications result from resource shortage rather than poor management or poor professional practice. That will of course require both to be able to demonstrate that those are not the explanations and to do so through the linkages available within the system at intermediate and national levels.

The need for the political arguments to be articulated locally poses a problem for any unified primary care in the context of existing local politics in the 1990s. Local government has been significantly marginalized within the system of central–local government relations in terms of formal government structures. Whether it should be revived is an open question, but if some effective system of legitimate local political representation is required then it seems to offer the only working model at present available. This raises another set of issues in relation to the Conservative government's reforms in the NHS and the response to them in terms of professional practice.

9

THE POLITICS OF THE NEW PRIMARY CARE

The concentration on professional and managerial issues in the previous chapters does not reflect acceptance of the widely expressed view that many problems experienced within the NHS would be more easily resolved if they could somehow be 'taken out of politics'. Nor does it reflect a wish to revert to the more distant past where professionals often played covert political roles at key points in the decision-making process. It rather reflects the view that politics are central to decisions about health care and that the political processes will operate more effectively within the NHS if the other aspects of provision are organized more coherently. This would require the system to move away from the current position where roles are confused and where location of responsibility and accountability are consequently problematic. The new market mechanisms were apparently introduced as a means of securing depoliticized decision making, moving responsibility and accountability for outcomes onto the local managerial and professional decision makers. In practice the market freedom to secure that transfer has not fully developed. The political implications of the decisions about care and their resource consequences have been too important to be left to market forces. This has led to a highly managed market, in which performance targets are set and priorities determined centrally, bringing politics into most areas of decision making, though in less transparent ways than before.

It is of course right and proper that such broad decisions should be taken centrally and be visible. The NHS is a major distributor, and politically more significant, a potential redistributor of a large volume of public resources (Le Grand 1982). This is closely involved with decisions about service and fundamentally concerned with the issues of equity and efficiency discussed earlier. Whatever its legitimacy, the pattern of intervention illustrates clearly both the difficulty of operating a pure market model in the context of the NHS, and of course the political significance of decisions taken every day by the managers and professionals working within the systems of care. This has led to a blurring of the boundaries between the levels within the NHS and the effective removal of the regional level and also between the boundaries of the different roles being played at each level. This has brought understandable disquiet among managers who, in applying central directives may appear to be exercising their local discretion and acting in political roles, and among professionals whose clinical judgement appears to be at fault when politically directed resource constraints restrict their exercise of discretion.

It has also led to a situation in which local ability to respond to particular circumstances, whether of constraint or of opportunity, is inhibited by the absence of a local politics to legitimize the exercise of discretion. The issue of local health care politics has been a long-running debate within the NHS with proposals to place health care within the existing local government structure rejected in 1946 and in the course of a number of subsequent reviews. It is worth re-visiting that debate and exploring the issues involved in light of the changes that have occurred in both local government and the NHS. It is particularly appropriate to do so in the context of a primary care-led NHS. A prime justification for that leading position is the relationship enjoyed with patients in primary care and the scope for new models of both direct and indirect democratic participation in the community setting.

FORMAL POLITICAL PROCESSES

It may be objected that there is already provision for the exercise of political roles within the organization of local health care. The NHS trusts and the health authorities (HAs) involve a small number of non-executive directors appointed by the Secretary of State. This has been an area of some political controversy, with the Labour party arguing that these appointments were politically motivated and engineered to secure local approval for national government policies. This argument assumes somewhat greater force in a context where one party is in office for a very long time, avoiding the more conventional swings and roundabouts of politi-cal appointments that would normally produce mixed board membership. Two other factors are perhaps more important than any charge of party bias in appointments. One is that those appointed owe their appointment, and are formally responsible to, the Secretary of State and not to the people of the locality in which they operate. The other is that many of those appointed seem to be chosen for their managerial skills and experience rather than their representative capacities. This is compounded in its effect when non-executives are drawn, as is often the case, from the private sector where the division of labour involved in the traditional public sector ethos does not apply.

That division of labour needs to be clarified if managers are to avoid being seen as the instrument of political will, rather than as the interpreters of that will into effective local opportunities for clinicians and associated professionals. Theoretically, within the traditional public service model, managers and professionals work together to make best use of limited resources within established political guidelines about priorities. They also offer advice to politicians during the decision-making process. If political guidelines impose unacceptable constraints on professional action, there is opportunity within the decision making processes for that issue to be addressed. Where it cannot be resolved at the operational level there are opportunities for professionals to engage in debate at higher levels within the system using both the professional service hierarchy and the more public route through their own representative structures. A similar argument may be applied to managers, although the basis of their legitimacy in arguing for alternative action is much more limited than that accorded to the professions. Nonetheless there is a case for management views to be heard, and mechanisms for doing so, about both policy and its implementation, if only to avoid failures in practice. There is also a growing movement towards management achieving professional status in its own right and developing its own patterns of professional organization and legitimacy to match those of the established clinical professions.

These mechanisms have experienced great strain during the recent period of accelerated reform in the NHS and none of the present structures provides an obvious model of political organization within which to accommodate the idea of a unified primary care system. Since the late 1970s traditional local government has been significantly marginalized within the framework of central–local government relations in both formal and informal terms. Local taxing and spending capacities have been curtailed and the framework of services altered in ways that match the changes in health care. New roles have been adopted by local authorities in relation to economic development and urban regeneration, but they do not replace those functions that have been lost. What local government has retained is its legitimizing system of local representation that seems to offer the only available working model if such a basis of legitimacy is accepted as being necessary within the NHS and within primary care.

Two approaches are available to take advantage of that model. One is to transfer the local delivery of NHS services, or at least primary care services, to the existing local authorities. That would meet the need for a single organization bringing together the varied services discussed in the last chapter. More importantly it would bring an immediate clarification of political responsibility in relation to local health care. The party political processes already in place would provide a focus for local policy making about health and related services, and at the same time provide the basis for testing popular rejection or support for such policies at elections. Political representation would also provide a mechanism for extending politics into the more detailed aspects of service provision, allowing for direct mutual feedback between the politics of policy and implementation. Adoption of this approach would raise a number of issues. It would add a political dimension to the relationship between the levels of decision making within the NHS, allowing a different kind of debate about local policy divergence. It would create potential conflict between national and local level, each claiming popular legitimacy for their decisions. Fundamental to that conflict would be the issue of resources, how much should be spent on health care and who should decide both the volume and the direction of spending. Finally there would no doubt be great professional concern about political intervention in what are currently regarded as purely professional decisions, though recent developments have already weakened the professional position and this argument.

On the question of political conflict those recent developments suggest difficulties for this model of reform. In all sectors it seems that the years since the early 1980s have involved a process of removing, or greatly weakening, intermediate levels of political decision. The need for local diversity to reflect genuine and legitimate local differences is accepted, but the machinery being devised to reflect this need involves extensive devolution with the autonomous small provider unit, or the individual patient, becoming the focus of decision. The problem for this model of service delivery is that capacities differ enormously in terms of the ability of people to be effectively involved in decisions. Also there is a tendency for the consequences of individual decision too easily to become the basis for shifts in national policy. The intermediate politics allow for an aggregation of popular interests at levels that reflect common social and economic factors and that can be sensitive to the distributive implications of policies and their implementation. The need for that element within the system remains, or its formal absence is met by a range of less satisfactory alternatives, some of which have been discussed earlier.

The resource question could be dealt with by a system of shared funding as is already the case with other expensive public services like education. There would be political tensions between centre and locality in some cases, but that is entirely appropriate in a service that recognizes that some local diversity is necessary. At least in this context local people would be able to react to decisions through a process that gives them much more legitimate influence than when they are seeking to influence decisions that are left to managers and professionals or to individual experience of professional care. The possibility of local political intervention in professional action would also create difficulties, not so much for social workers who already experience its effects, but for health professionals who do not. It would be more easily resolved, however, in a setting where such interventions arose in the context of joint professional working and where local policy already reflected the political input often missing in the present system. In principle of course it would be no different from the current position where members of parliament are prone to take up individual issues as part of the dialogue around central policy making. The key difference would lie in the immediacy of the contact and the greater ability at the local level to shift policy and practice in light of experience, and involve all the role players in such a shift.

Such a change would mark a radical break with the historical tendency to weaken local government and seems most unlikely to be introduced in the present political climate, though a change of government could alter that prospect. Another solution would be to create an elected health authority to serve alongside the existing local government, sharing the same basis of legitimacy for its decisions. This could involve independent local taxing powers although the same arguments would apply in relation to control of public spending as currently do in relation to local government.

Given this constraint an alternative would be for an elected authority to work within the context of centrally determined and devolved budgets. This would weaken the influence of such a locally elected authority by depriving it of taxing powers, but it is little different in practice from the present situation in local government and health care. The rhetoric is rich with comments about local autonomy in the use of central resources but the reality is highly constrained. The important gain would be policy decisions and resultant implementation being undertaken by bodies responsible and accountable to their local populations in visible and legitimate ways.

These would not need to be large representative bodies on the model of current local authorities. Indeed small elected memberships might serve to focus political attention at the policy level locally leaving the questions of detailed delivery to be dealt with on the patch through different processes. These more local issues lend themselves to more direct forms of public involvement, particularly when the policy context locally has become much more transparent. This could allow for the development of participation properly geared to the level of decision and improve the overall flow of information, which is essential for effective participation at each of the levels involved.

PATIENT POWER AND CITIZEN CONTROL

In the context of participation it is essential first to establish the difference between involvement as patient and involvement as citizen. This is very clear in the development of the reforms where the *Patient's Charter* (Department of Health 1995b) forms the NHS version of the more general *Citizen's Charter* (Cabinet Office 1991) programme. The charter follows the consumerist argument that lies at the basis of the quasi-market in health care and accords the patient a number of specified rights, and a longer list of expectations, against which they can assess their experience of health care. Rights are specified in relation to GP services and include a right to be registered with a GP, and to change that registration easily and quickly. Patients have a right to information about available services, to be offered or be able to ask for health checks, and to be prescribed appropriate medication where necessary (Department of Health 1995a). The Conservative government urged practices to establish their own charters, and many are doing so, but the items involved do not stray further into matters of professional judgement nor of practice policies in relation to priorities and developments. The charter does provide the patient/consumer with some leverage after they have received treatment if they feel that some aspect within the charter guidelines has been inadequately met. This puts clear limits on the timing, character and scope of patient rights, moving them into the area of complaints, rather than into proactive involvement with practice policies and decisions. Of course the existence of the charter may influence patient and professional attitudes and so change the character of their interactions in the surgery and more broadly in the running of practices. In this it would be aided and abetted by the widespread media interest in matters medical and to do with health, which provides some patients with a capacity in terms of knowledge that they previously did not possess.

Empowerment of individual patients is a good thing perhaps, but falls short of the wider role that they might play collectively as citizens in policy development in relation to their primary care. This debate has a longer history, but the recent emphasis on managerialism and efficiency in much health service reform has tended to keep it as a marginal issue. The reforms of 1974 concentrated in this way but did include the somewhat belated decision to create Community Health Councils (CHCs). Their membership was drawn from local authorities and the voluntary sector and they were given a limited though important role, in representing the interests of local people in the context of health care decisions. They had to be consulted about some decisions and in their early years this led to a concentration on secondary care where the impact of decisions about hospital provision was highly visible, and the decision process one in which formal participation by the CHC was possible. Their other main role was in acting as advocate to individuals experiencing difficulties with, or making complaints about, their health care. On both fronts they were limited in what they could do by having very few staff and being responsible for quite large geographical areas.

The CHCs can be seen as the NHS response to the wide concern at that time with issues about citizen participation in the public services more generally. Since their creation in the mid-1970s a wide variety of such programmes with varied levels of official support and widely different conceptions of the proper role of citizens in public services have been developed. In the early years this was reflected in a variety of projects seeking to create community-based health groups, councils or partnerships, aimed at playing a more proactive and perhaps directive role in the development of health care policy and with wider aims consistent with the new public health movement which emerged later in the 1980s and 1990s (Ashton and Seymour 1988). These efforts reflected the general popularity of community development as the basis for a change in the distribution of power and influence in relation to public policy, especially in the more deprived areas where service quality was seen as being less satisfactory.

Primary care has not been a major focus for these kinds of developments, partly because of its quite separate organization and the formal employment status of GPs, and partly because of levels of satisfaction with its performance. There were some early efforts, for example, to establish practice based patients' groups, but this never developed into a widespread movement. This reflects the character of individual patient care and the difficulty of engaging patients as citizens in wider concerns, and of course the unwillingness of many professionals to accept such a broadening of role in any case. The National Patients' Association reflects this difficulty at a more general level, not easily engaging members and not being markedly influential in the broad debate, nor at the local delivery of health care (Boaden *et al.* 1981). When the issues of care move beyond the individual level, engaging political processes and questions of citizen rather than patient participation, there is a strong tendency for the formal political processes to be seen as taking over, distancing the public in the process.

The more recent Conservative government reforms in the NHS have made the situation more difficult in creating formal structures and processes within which public participation has no obvious place in the citizen sense. At the same time government has recognized the need to legitimize the system with some elements of popular participation, though it has not been willing to introduce direct elections as the obvious basis for doing so. The result has been a good deal of exhortation around the issue of public participation, and a wide development of experiments to engage the public in some decisions about health care.

The exhortation has come almost entirely around the purchasing side of the new market model of health care, drawing primary care firmly into the net as a significant part of that process. The implication that purchasing decisions dictate provision and imply no need for direct public participation on the provider side needs closer examination. The evidence is still not clear about this in relation to the purchasing of secondary care, though it is evident that the annual purchasing decision in which the public is involved betrays a limited view of effective public participation in a dynamic continuing relationship like that between primary and secondary care. The formal commissioning process provides an ideal focus for participatory opportunities, but the dynamics which follow that process are also important and a much more difficult context for wide involvement. In relation to primary care itself, there is no commissioning process involved so that some form of participation in the provider setting is essential for citizen involvement. This does not currently appear to be on the agenda of debate, except in so far as HAs are beginning to grapple with their relationships both with primary care and with their local populations.

In terms of the commissioning role, the many initiatives reflect a wide range of approaches familiar from earlier efforts in other areas of public policy making with new additions of more recent origin. Prominent in the rhetoric, and in the practice, are a number of techniques for consulting with large groups of people or with representative samples drawn from such groups. They range from engagement with specific groups interested in health care to attempts to engage more broadly with whole populations. In terms of technique they include public meetings, which are a good way to tell people rather than hear from them about developments (Boaden *et al.* 1982). They include opinion polling and sample surveys, which secure representative sampling of opinion, but often at the expense of being unable to ask the difficult questions involved in complex policies like primary care. That problem is overcome in some cases by the use of focus groups of various kinds, which allow complex and interactive debate, but of course only involve small numbers of people and considerable expense to maintain on any frequent basis.

All of these efforts go some way towards 'tackling the democratic deficit in health' (Cooper *et al.* 1995). They mark a beginning to the difficult process of widening the public role, but they have occurred in a piecemeal way, within the conventions of the existing political process, and without much debate about the appropriate role of the public in a complex and highly professionalized service. This becomes much clearer if one starts at a more basic level and examines some of the discussions that have arisen in other areas of public policy. Planning is an area where public participation was a relatively early statutory requirement, but where the evidence suggests there was great difficulty in establishing an ongoing process of participation in situations where politicians, professionals and public might clash (Boaden *et al.* 1981). This was particularly the case at the level of strategic decisions, especially where implementation lay in the future when circumstances and attitudes might have changed. This reflects the realities of the political process and the short term character of much decision making even within the formal political processes. It certainly applies in a resource-costly service such as the NHS.

The difficulties in this task become clearer if one looks at an early conceptualization of public participation in the context of planning. Arnstein's (1969) ladder of citizen participation provides a useful starting point for our discussion. This involved consideration of participation and its implications for the citizens in relation to their power and influence within the system (see Figure 9.1).

If the rhetoric of current efforts, and the character of the initiatives just considered, are placed on the ladder it becomes immediately clear that much effort has remained on the lower rungs. Certainly it is difficult to see any initiative that falls within the area of citizen power, though it is possible that there may be examples of partnership at very local levels. Therapy and manipulation are not obviously part of the current initiatives, but informing and consulting the public loom very large in most examples. Decision makers are not formally bound by the inputs made by the public, and failure to respond does not easily lead to further public influence because of the lack of democratic processes. The CHCs are the one formal vehicle in the system but only enjoy the right to be consulted about certain kinds of decisions. Other groups may be influential over particular issues where their political impact can be

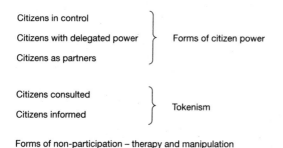

Figure 9.1 Levels of citizen participation
Adapted from: Arnstein (1969).

mobilized in other ways, though they are unlikely to enjoy such influence over a wide range of issues. Indeed they often gain their higher place only by accepting more modest levels of participation on other issues. Participation is a costly process and resources are limited both within the system and among the potential participants. Development of the resource base for citizen power would be an expensive decision for government and equally so for any group not accorded a formal role within the process of health care decision making.

Reverting to the systems model it is very evident that the lower rungs of the ladder have a significant place in the creation, cultivation and expression of support for the existing system. When it comes to questions of need and demand the ladder hardly applies. Certainly primary care individualizes the process of participation, placing the onus on the patient to take up and negotiate the care on offer. The idea of collective citizen input to the process is then quite remote with arguments about individual patient's rights and professional decision making looming large to challenge the legitimacy of wider involvement.

This is a pity as the current model of general practice offers an excellent context within which to provide for participation. The population involved is not too large for effective interaction, being formally registered with the practice and so identifiable, displaying considerable stability over time and in the main having some direct experience of using the service. All these are ingredients that might be expected to motivate participants and on which to build an effective continuing system of participation. In such a context it should be possible to move people further up the participatory ladder, but of course this becomes a matter of will on their part and on that of the professionals involved. Any move towards such higher levels of participation by one group of course disturbs the position of others. Professionals might feel threatened and activists might gain advantage over less active participants in terms of service. These are issues that have been addressed in other areas of public service such as housing where housing associations and cooperatives have shown considerable success and where the rationale for greater public participation is no greater than in health care.

Further development would of course depend on much greater clarity about the range of decisions being made in practice, and about the proper roles that might be expected for different actors in that situation. The analogy with school governors is not inappropriate, with a real shift of power away from the professionals in respect of some decisions about the running and direction of schools. Would such a pattern be possible in primary care? Certainly not while the employment structure remains as it is in general practice but that should perhaps be the issue for debate.

What seems clear from the discussion is that the creation of a two tier primary care system with a single county-wide authority, and patch based interdisciplinary delivery, would together provide a good setting for linking the public to both policy and implementation. The former would provide an ideal vehicle for an elected authority. The latter would provide an ideal context for the effective use of most of the techniques involved in direct public participation in public services. The combination would secure a responsive and accountable structure that the current market mechanisms seem unlikely to deliver.

10

CONCLUSIONS

Underlying the discussion throughout this book has been the central importance of the goal of optimal health for all and the importance to its achievement of an effective, equitable and efficient health care system. At the same time examination of the long history of development of health care confirms that by itself such a system is unlikely to deliver the goal of optimal health. The earliest developments in public health stress the importance of other factors, and the significance of government intervention in a wide range of areas indirectly relevant to the state of the public health. Subsequent development strengthens that message and the reforms of the 1940s followed Beveridge in seeking to introduce a coherent and connected system across the range of government services. The British National Health Service was the instrument of direct government involvement in health care, but was to be developed in parallel with reformed intervention in all sectors. Development since 1948 emphasizes the difficulty of implementing such an integrated approach, and the elusive nature of optimal health, with the results of reform varying widely between sectors of health care, areas of the country and groups in society. Advances in medicine, in standards of care and in public expectations have in any case moved the optimal goal and have made its delivery ever more difficult and expensive. Taken together, the successes and the failures since 1948 serve to underline both the importance of connections in achieving improved public health, and the difficulty of making them.

This explains the theme of making connections that runs through the text and is now being openly advocated in formal government documents (NHS Executive 1996; Secretary of State 1996b). Apart from the overarching importance of the connection with the past, three sets of connections were identified as being of importance: first, as was already clear by 1860, the connections between the economic and social conditions that influence health and the range of government activity to influence and mitigate those factors in favour of public health; second, the connections within the health care system itself, both between levels and between sectors, in what has emerged as an ever more complex matrix of provision; third, the relationships within each sector of care, between the professions involved, between them and the politicians and managers, and between these different provider groups and the people who receive health care. All of these are relevant in primary care and their significance is increased by the most recent Conservative government policies, which accord the sector a central role in the future development of the NHS.

Examination of reform over 50 years in the NHS, and in related government activity, confirms that the significance of these connections is recognized, but that making them effectively is a complex and difficult task. The failure to do so stems in part from the legacy of the past with its fragmented structure, both in health care itself and in the context within which it is provided. Successive reforms have addressed that issue, but integration has proved difficult, partly due to the institutionalized divisions involved and partly to their reinforcement by a range of entrenched interests with extensive influence, if not power, in the decision-making process.

The most recent Conservative reforms confirm the need for connection, and the perceived limitations of the traditional reform process in making those connections. In terms of process they illustrate much more directive decision making on the part of central government, with professional interests being relatively marginalized in the process. This accounts for a widely held professional perception of reform being imposed rather than agreed, and may explain at least some of the limitations apparent in the take up and implementation of reform. Change in the process of reform has been associated with significant substantive changes in the NHS generally and in primary care in particular. In terms of relationships between levels and sectors, the internal market has been established and is changing intersectoral influence by providing new mechanisms for making connections. Within primary care, the new GP contract, fundholding and parallel changes in the provision of community care, have begun to change professional and institutional relationships. These have been associated with much greater central direction through performance targets and publication of information, and by the Citizen's Charter movement according formal rights to patients (Cabinet Office 1991).

Such reforms appear to have a radical edge, but examination of the scope of change suggests that their impact has been more limited in primary care than the rhetoric might suggest. Certainly changes have occurred, and in some cases been extensive and radical, but their perceived imposition may have led to an exaggerated impression of actual change in practice. Evidence about innovation, and more importantly, about its diffusion, especially around fundholding suggests that it has been limited. The small number of radical practices who have made significant changes are outnumbered by the many who have engaged more modestly with the opportunities provided by having their own budgets. In any case, much of the change has been around the area of purchasing secondary care, embracing a wider range of general practices involved in experiments in commissioning as an alternative approach. This is important in beginning to change the intersectoral relations within health care, but in relation to the delivery of primary care itself change seems to have been more limited. There have been developments but they reflect the limited pattern of innovation always present in general practice, rather than the extended change that reform might have been expected to encourage.

Examination of this record of change, together with the messages of history, suggests the need for a more radical analysis. Systems theory confirms the significance of connections, but also suggests some of the complexities that might be limiting the effect of reform. Some reform of process has been introduced, but into a structure of primary care that remains as fragmented and as varied as ever. Implementation of the new processes is being left to professionals trained in quite traditional ways, often not well adapted to meet the demands of traditional primary care, let alone to meet the demands generated by the reforms. The failure to address this combination of structural and cultural limitations has, it is argued, resulted in sharp limitations being placed on the extent of reform.

These two aspects of primary care were addressed in earlier chapters. On the cultural side an assessment was made of the nature of primary care and the professional mix involved in its provision given the new roles that might be involved in establishing a primary care-led NHS. That discussion suggested the possibility of significant change in the balance of professional activity, but also highlighted wider roles that will be required of some participants within primary care. Research as the basis for evidence based practice, audit and research and development, and the wide advocacy role involved in assessment of, and action around, health need and health are all emerging in the Conservative government agenda (Secretary of State 1996a, 1996b). All are new to primary care and all require skills and resources that are not obviously forthcoming in the immediate future. The multiprofessional team that is appearing within primary care needs to become an interprofessional team, with specialist development being introduced to provide appropriate services and support for generalist colleagues. More radically it was suggested that there is a case for looking at primary care in new ways, developing a primary care profession who share common training that links the divergent elements of the disparate training enjoyed by the professions currently involved.

In either case developments of this kind imply a clear case for a radical overhaul of professional training for primary care, again an issue recognized in the latest government documents (Secretary of State 1996c). This involves a number of elements. Substantively it requires a new curriculum in which the basis of the wider range of relevant skills is embodied in the early subjects of study and experiences offered in training. The in-depth study deemed essential for specialist careers in acute care needs to give way to a breadth of study that recognizes the complexity of the community and family context within which primary care is provided. This will involve the clinical sciences, but also those social sciences that provide understanding of the source of much ill-health, and of the character of effective provision to deal with it. Such breadth would provide the basis for a new primary care profession, but would also have great benefit in terms of more effective interprofessional awareness than is provided by the current divided system of training. In any event, that interprofessional aspect needs to be built into the educational process with shared learning becoming the hallmark of initial as well as of continuing professional education.

Institutionally such changes will require the professions and the training organizations, colleges and universities to make significant changes themselves. In professional terms this will be difficult as any such changes strike at the core of established professional identity, which is based on differences rather than similarities. In direct educational terms it is less problematic in the sense that such changes readily fit the developing model of higher education with its looser structures and more interdisciplinary focus. Some of this change is already apparent in changes in nursing and in the changes being introduced into undergraduate medicine, but the need is for training driven by the needs of primary care, rather than for professionals trained for other careers then having to adapt to primary care. Greater experience of primary care settings during training will have some benefit, but if it continues within the narrow bounds of traditional specialisms then it will have limited impact on the new situation (Secretary of State 1996c).

Professional changes of this kind would have beneficial effect, but their impact would be greatly enhanced by the introduction of more fundamental change in the structures for primary care delivery. It was suggested that these might take the form of larger area-wide primary care organizations able to take a broad perspective about health need and resource allocation. Their service delivery functions would be devolved to smaller localities but this too could be managed more directly and effectively within a single coherent organization. The division of labour between professionals and managers and politicians would be clearer and policy making more transparent. This would allow for improved links between levels of decision making, creating a context for easier implementation of change. In terms of professional education, certainly postgraduate and continuing education, such organizations would provide a context in which experiential education, and informal professional development, could be met in an interdisciplinary, operational setting. The increased scale and vertical links involved in a new structure would facilitate wider educational development, allowing participation at different levels and providing a resource base more adequate to the needs involved. The wider needs of the Primary Health Care Team could also be better considered in a multidisciplinary context, which would itself provide formal and informal shared learning opportunities as well.

More directly in relation to service development a more coherent structure would allow new developments, avoid the awkward inter-agency relationships that currently have to be overcome to achieve them, and above all provide clear links between levels of concern that are relevant to primary care. It would allow sensitive resource allocation at a more strategic level, but one in which dialogue with localities would be part of the normal processes of primary care delivery. Such a context would offer a much more coherent opportunity for the public to become involved, in relation to policy making as well as in the more direct details of their own care. If the former required the machinery of elections to give it legitimacy then this would also provide a context in which that could be organized.

CONTINUING REFORM

The suggestions being made here for further changes in primary care need to be seen in relation to the proposals for continuing reform outlined in a series of relatively recent government documents (Secretary of State 1996a, 1996b, 1996c). These follow a period of government consultation with a range of groups and though they reveal an intention to continue the process of change, the Conservative government accepts that 'there is considerable interest in trying out these ideas, there was no enthusiasm for moving directly to any or all of these options without careful exploration first and no enthusiasm for forced change' (Secretary of State 1996b: para. 2.6). In terms of process, government is committed to 'change by consent and consultation involving volunteers' and to 'pilots with proper evaluation' (Secretary of State 1996b: para. 1.5). This change of approach seems partly to reflect the uncertainty of politics in a long pre-election period and partly acknowledgement of the reaction of the professions to the recent reforms. In the case of general practice, this is reinforced by reported stress among GPs and difficulties in recruitment to general practice, which are being attributed to the impact of reform and the processes that it involves. For those who hoped for a period of consolidation after the spate of reform, this changed approach to the process must be welcome. For those who think that further reform, or at least greatly extended adoption of existing good practice, is necessary, it may be seen as a sign that the Conservative government is unwilling to tackle the difficult political and resource questions involved in a more radical future.

How to achieve necessary change is the important issue, as examination of the current government proposals in many ways confirms the analysis offered earlier about the deficiencies in the current system of primary care. The government proposals for delivering the future confirm their recognition of the importance of many of the linkages discussed. The theme of partnership is very strong, between levels within primary care and among the professions involved with a clear need for changes in professional education, emphasizing its relevance to primary care and the importance of interprofessional training (Secretary of State 1996c). So too are the difficult questions around resource allocation and the current negative discrimination implicit in a system where some aspects of resourcing are not related to levels of local need (Secretary of State 1996c: paras 5.5, 5.6). The importance of management in primary care, particularly where change remains a priority, is also highlighted, contrasting somewhat with the pressure to reduce management costs within the acute sector (Secretary of State 1996c). Better organization of primary care is acknowledged as being necessary, but there is no hint of the more general reorganization being suggested here. Indeed in the latest White Paper it is made clear that 'the ambitions set out in this document do not rely on further radical change. They are rooted in the best of current practice' (Secretary of State 1996c: 7). Their widespread adoption, which appears to be the aim, would of course be a radical change.

There is some overlap between the detailed recommendations from the Conservative government around each of these issues and those discussed earlier but it is in the broad approach to dealing with agreed limitations and failings within primary care that the differences emerge. For the government the future is to be delivered through research, consultation, pilot experimentation and voluntary participation and improved information and dissemination (Secretary of State 1996c). The imposed tone and character of recent reform has gone, and the Secretary of State is explicit about the need for professional consent and approval for further change, certainly in relation to general practice. This hints at a reversion to an older style of reform and to what might be characterized as the conventional incremental approach to development within the NHS. This has not been shown to produce radical change, even over extended periods, or done much to remove the inverse care law in relation to primary care that lies at the root of some of the current proposals. It accepts a model of professionally directed development, seeing GPs as the pivotal group in primary care, and proposes health authority (HA) and government support to facilitate the process of change, with limited resource allocations to steer development and stimulate experiment and change. This approach has obvious short term attractions, involving limited spending and giving government some control over the direction of change. In the longer term, wider adoption of any changes will involve changing the less willing professionals, and reform that has been driven by financial support or incentive may prove expensive when wider adoption is being considered. Resources are needed to facilitate change, but they would be best spent on creating corporate recognition of, and capacity for, change rather than facilitating individual opportunity. In a climate of perceived autonomy it could be that everyone will need to undertake their own research and development to reflect the uniqueness of their own practice. In the more uniform evidence-based primary care that is intended, where such uniqueness is not perhaps the key characteristic, a different approach to change would seem to be called for.

The Conservative government's choice of approach seems to reflect several intentions. One is the evident wish to get rid of the present variation in quality within primary care. Another is to assist the professions to put their own house in order, though at the same time to encourage the culture of individual autonomy, which inhibits them from doing that. A third is the need to limit cost rises creating a very tight financial climate in which to introduce change. A fourth is the wish to sustain the general market philosophy of the recent reforms, and the idea of patient choice, both of which are seen to require a plurality of modes of provision.

Few would argue with the first of these, indeed it lies at the core of the argument outlined here. The others do not at once seem the most obvious ways to achieve such equity, certainly not within a context of resource constraint. Examination of current evidence suggests that there is much variety within the existing system and that it is not often congruent with the different patterns of need for primary care evident both socially and geographically. The variety stems rather from the current highly fragmented structure of care, and the culture of professional autonomy and separation that is characteristic of much practice. Such evidence suggests that plurality and diversity are not obvious routes to equity, nor that voluntary compliance, which gives providers an effective veto on reform, is consistent with the wide dissemination of best practice and the adoption of change.

One problem with the proposed approach is its dominant concern with a traditional and narrow view of primary care as general practice, which may be extended by GPs in voluntary ways. This limits the view taken about change and serves to emphasize the importance of GP approval of any package of further changes. If there is a current crisis within general practice such an approach is likely to produce short term problems given the length of training involved. The wider view of primary care taken here, and emerging in some Royal College of General Practitioners (RCGP) discussion, should prompt the question as to whether there are other solutions to the shortage of GPs (Mathie 1997). The need is to organize, train and recruit with a future primary care in mind, and one in which a new division of labour may change the role of the GP and other professionals involved. This may bring a reduced need for conventional GPs or a significant reduction in the length of training currently involved. Extended training for general practice that is being proposed should be considered in this context and the suitability of the full initial medical education as a basis for such postgraduate training considered. Such an approach might also change the rigid criteria often applied during initial recruitment, allowing access to the career of those more suited to the nature of future primary care.

Inevitably in a sense, in deciding to approach reform in this way, the Conservative government has conditioned all other aspects of current policy. The detail of that policy recognizes the diagnosis offered earlier. What it fails to do is legislate for how change will be introduced effectively, and more importantly how it will be diffused successfully to meet the criteria of cost-effective and equitable care. This is a pity because events may have created an opportunity for more radical change of the kind proposed here. The recent reforms seemed to have broken the traditional mould in terms of how the NHS is organized, the relative influence of the different groups within it, and in particular have recognized the central role of primary care. Together with changes in the reform process itself a context has been created in which the need for further reform is clearly apparent and, despite talk of the desirability of a period of consolidation, may be possible. These contradictory attitudes stem from the fact that the reform process itself has challenged traditional patterns of influence. Most strikingly, in common with other public services, the powerful position of the dominant professional interests has been challenged. This has significantly divided opinion within the medical profession, some doctors resenting any change that they perceive as being improperly imposed, others welcoming the new opportunities that reform has brought, even where they may not approve the way in which it has been introduced.

Capitalizing on the potential created by reform does not involve kicking the professionals while they are down. Nor should it involve a reversion to a context where they appear to be the key determinants of future change. It should involve a debate within a wider primary care about the goals that all seem to accept, but also about ways in which they might be achieved given the traditional failure to meet them. This book is offered as a contribution to that debate.

BIBLIOGRAPHY

Abel-Smith, B. (1960). *A History of the Nursing Profession*. London: Heinemann.

Alford, R.R. (1969). *Bureaucracy and Participation*. Chicago, IL: Rand McNally.

Allan, P. and Jolly, M. (eds) (1987). *Nursing, Midwifery and Health Visiting since 1900*. London: Faber.

Allsop, J. (1984). *Health Policy and the National Health Service*. London: Longman.

Arnstein, S.R. (1969). A ladder of citizen participation. *Journal of the American Institute of Planners*, 35(4), 216–24.

Ashton, J. and Seymour, H. (1988). *The New Public Health*. Buckingham: Open University Press.

Audit Commission (1993). *Practices Made Perfect: The Role of the Family Health Services Authority*. London: HMSO.

Audit Commission (1996a). *Fundholding Facts: A Digest of Information About Practices Within the Scheme During the First Five Years*. London: HMSO.

Audit Commission (1996b). *What the Doctor Ordered: A Study of GP Fundholders in England and Wales*. London: HMSO.

Barr, H. (1994). *Perspectives on Shared Learning*. London: CAIPE.

Barr, H. and Waterton, S. (1996). *Interprofessional Education in Health and Social Care in the United Kingdom*. London: CAIPE.

Beveridge, Sir W. (1942). *Social Insurance and Allied Services*. London: HMSO.

Birch, S. and Maynard, A. (1987). Regional distribution of family practitioner services: implications for National Health Service equity and efficiency. *Journal of the Royal College of General Practitioners*, 37, 537–9.

Bligh, J. and Parsell, G. (1995). Shaking up the class system. *Health Service Journal*, 105, (5448), 23.

Boaden, N. (1971). *Urban Policy Making*. Cambridge: Cambridge University Press.

Boaden, N., Goldsmith, M., Hampton, W. and Stringer, P. (1981). Planning and participation in practice. *Progress in Planning*, 13, 1–102.

Boaden, N., Goldsmith, M., Hampton, W. and Stringer, P. (1982). *Public Participation in Local Services*. London: Longman.

Booth, C. (1889–1903). *Life and Labour of the People of London*. London: Macmillan.

Bradshaw, J. (1972). The taxonomy of social need. In G. McLachlan (ed.) *Problems and Progress in Medical Care*. London: Nuffield Provincial Hospitals Trust.

British Medical Association (1965). *Charter for the Family Doctor Service*. London: BMA.

Cabinet Office (1991). *The Citizen's Charter: Raising the Standard*, Cm 1599. London: HMSO.

Cain, P., Hyde, P. and Hawkins, E. (eds) (1995). *Community Nursing; Dimensions and Dilemmas*. London: Arnold.

Clare, A. and Corney, R.H. (1982). *Social Work and Primary Health Care*. London: Academic Press.

Cooper, L., Coote, A., Davies, A. and Jackson, C. (1995). *Voices Off: Tackling the Democratic Deficit in Health*. London: Institute of Public Policy Research.

Damant, M., Martin, C. and Openshaw, S. (1994). *Practice Nursing: Stability and Change*. London: Mosby.

Department of Health (1995a). *Statistical Bulletins: Statistics for general medical practitioners in England, 1984–1994*. London: Department of Health.

Department of Health (1995b). *Patient's Charter*. London: HMSO.

Department of Health (1995c). *Health and Personal Social Services Statistics for England*. London: HMSO.

Duggan, M. (1995). *Primary Health Care: A Prognosis*. London: Institute of Public Policy Research.

Easton, D. (1965). *Systems Analysis of Political Life*. New York: Wiley.

Etzioni, A. (1969). *The Semi-Professions and Their Organization*. New York: Free Press.

Flynn, R. (1992). *Structures of Control in Health Management*. London: Routledge and Kegan Paul.

Fraser, D. (1973). *The Evolution of the British Welfare State*. London: Macmillan.

Fry, J. (1988). *General Practice and Primary Health Care, 1940s–1980s*. London: Nuffield Provincial Hospitals Trust.

Fry, J. (1993). *General Practice: The Facts*. Oxford: Radcliffe Medical Press.

General Medical Council Education Committee (1993). *Tomorrow's Doctors*. London: General Medical Council.

Gilbert, B. (1966). *The Evolution of National Insurance*. London: Joseph.

Glennerster, H., Matsaganis, M., Owens, P. and Hancock, S. (1994). *Implementing GP Fundholding: A Wild Card or a Winning Hand?* Buckingham: Open University Press.

Goldsmith, M. (1980). *Politics, Planning and the City*. London: Hutchinson.

Gordon, P. and Hadley, J. (1996). *Extending Primary Care: Polyclinics,*

Resource Centres, Hospitals at Home. Oxford: Radcliffe Medical Press.

Griffiths, R. (1983). *NHS Management Enquiry.* London: DHSS.

Griffiths, R. (1988). *Community Care: Agenda for Action.* London: HMSO.

Hacking, J. (1996). Weight watchers. *Health Services Journal,* 106 (5501), 28–30.

Hadley, R. and Forster, D. (1993). *Doctors as Managers: Experiences in the Front Line of the NHS.* Harlow: Longman.

Hadley, R. and Young, K. (1990). *Creating a Responsive Public Service.* London: Harvester Wheatsheaf.

Hall, P., Land, H., Parker, R. and Webb, A. (1975). *Change, Choice and Conflict in Social Policy.* London: Heinemann.

Hannay, D.A., Usherwood, T.P. and Platts, M. (1992). Practice organization before and after the new contract: a survey of general practices in Sheffield. *British Journal of General Practice,* 42, 517–20.

Harrison, S., Hunter, D. and Pollitt, C. (1990). *The Dynamics of British Health Policy.* London: Routledge and Kegan Paul.

Harrison, S. and Hunter, D.J. (1995). *Rationing Health Care.* London: Intitute of Public Policy Research.

Hart, J.T. (1971). The inverse care law. *The Lancet,* i, 405–12.

Hart, J.T. (1988). *A New Kind of Doctor: The General Practitioners Part in the Health of the Community.* London: Merlin Press.

Hay, J.R. (1975). *The Origins of the Liberal Welfare Reforms.* London: Macmillan.

Heath, I. (1995). *The Mystery of General Practice.* London: Nuffield Provincial Hospitals Trust.

Henry, S. and Pickersgill, D. (eds) (1995). *Making Sense of Fundholding.* Oxford: Radcliffe Medical Press.

Hirschman, A.O. (1970). *Exit, Voice and Loyalty.* Cambridge, MA: Harvard University Press.

Houle, C.O. (1980). *Continuing Learning in the Professions.* New York: Jossey-Bass.

Hunter, D. and Webster, C. (1992). Here we go again. *Health Services Journal,* 102 (5292), 26–7.

Huntington, J. (1981). *Social Work and General Medical Practice: Collaboration or Conflict?* London: Allen and Unwin.

Huntington, J. (1995). *Managing the Practice: Whose Business?* Oxford: Radcliffe Medical Press.

Inter-Departmental Committee on Physical Deterioration (1904). *Report.* London: HMSO.

Irvine, D. (1990). *Management for Quality in General Practice.* London: King's Fund Centre.

Irvine, D. (1993). General practice in the 1990s: a personal view on future development. *British Journal of General Practice,* 43, 121–8.

Itano, J.K., Williams, J., Deaton, M.D. and Oishi, N. (1991). Impact of a student interdisciplinary oncology team project. *Journal of Cancer Education,* 4(4), 219–26.

Johnson, N., Hasler, J., Toby, J. and Grant J. (1996a). Content of a trainer's report for summative assessment in general practice: views of trainers. *British Journal of General Practice*, 46, 135–9.

Johnson, N., Hasler, J., Toby, J. and Grant J. (1996b). Consensus minimum standards for use in a trainer's report for summative assessment in general practice. *British Journal of General Practice*, 46, 140–4.

Klein, R. (1989). *The Politics of the NHS* (2nd edn). London: Longman.

Klein, R. and Lewis, J. (1976). *The Politics of Consumer Representation: A Study of Community Health Councils*. London: Centre for Studies in Social Policy.

Leese, B. and Bosanquet, N. (1995a). Family doctors and change in practice strategy since 1986. *British Medical Journal*, 310, 705–8.

Leese, B. and Bosanquet, N. (1995b). Change in general practice and its effects on service provision in areas with different socioeconomic characteristics. *British Medical Journal*, 311, 546–50.

Le Grand, J. (1982). *The Strategy of Equality*. London: Allen and Unwin.

Le Grand, J. and Bartlett, W. (eds) (1994). *Quasi-Markets and Social Policy*. Basingstoke: Macmillan.

Lloyd, M., Webb, S. and Singh, S. (1995). *General Practitioners and the Community Care Reforms*. Royal Free Hospital School of Medicine, London: Department of General Practice.

McCormick, A., Fleming, D. and Charlton, J. (1995). *Morbidity Statistics From General Practice: Fourth National Study 1991–1992*. London: HMSO.

Mathie, A.G. (1997). *The Primary Care Workforce: A Descriptive Analysis*. London: Royal College of General Practioners.

Meads, G. (1996). *Future Options for General Practice*. Oxford: Radcliffe Medical Press.

Merrison, Sir Alec (Chairman) (1979). *Royal Commission on the National Health Service*, Cmnd 7615. London: HMSO.

National Audit Office (1992). *Nursing Education: Implementation of Project 2000 in England*. London: HMSO.

National Health Service Executive (1996). *Primary Care: The Future*. London: HMSO.

Noakes, J. (1992). The case for a primary health care authority. *British Journal of General Practice*, 308, 355–7.

Øvretveit, J. (1993). *Coordinating Community Care: Multi-Disciplinary Teams and Care Management*. Buckingham: Open University Press.

Pietroni, R. (1991). New strategies for higher professional education. *British Journal of General Practice*. 42, 294–6.

Pietroni, P. and Pietroni, C. (eds) (1996). *Innovation in Community Care and Primary Health: The Marylebone Experience*. London: Churchill Livingstone.

Pratt, J. (1995). *Practitioners and Practices: A Conflict of Values*. Oxford: Radcliffe Medical Press.

Resource Allocation Working Party (1976). *Sharing Resources for Health in England*. London: HMSO.

Robinson, R. and Le Grand, J. (eds) (1994). *Evaluating the NHS Reforms*. Newbury: Policy Journals.

Rowntree, B.S. (1901). *Poverty: A Study of Town Life*. London: Macmillan.

Royal College of General Practitioners (1985). *The Front Line of the Health Service*. London: RCGP.

Royal College of General Practitioners (1987). *Quality in General Practice*. London: RCGP.

Schön, D.A. (1983). *The Reflective Practitioner: How Professionals Think in Action*. New York: Harper Collins.

Secretary of State for Health (1992). *The Health of the Nation*. Cmnd 1986. London: HMSO.

Secretary of State for Health (1996a). *Choice and Opportunity. Primary Care: The Future*. London: HMSO.

Secretary of State for Health (1996b). *The National Health Service: A Service with Ambitions*, Cmnd 3425. London: HMSO.

Secretary of State for Health (1996c). *Primary Care: Delivering the Future*. London: HMSO.

Seebohm Committee on Local Authority and Allied Social Services (1968). *Report*. Cmnd 2703. London: HMSO.

Shakespeare, H., Tucker, W. and Northover, J. (1989). *Report of a National Survey of Interprofessional Education in Primary Health Care*. London: CAIPE.

Smith, L.F.P. (1994). Higher professional training in general practice: provision of master's degree courses in the United Kingdom in 1993. *British Medical Journal*. 308, 1679–82.

Starfield, B. (1992). *Primary Care: Concept, Evaluation and Policy*. New York: Oxford University Press.

Stocking, B. (1985). *Initiative and Inertia: Case Studies in the NHS*. London: Nuffield Provincial Hospitals Trust.

Titmuss, R. (1950). *Problems of Social Policy*. London: HMSO.

Tomlinson, B. (1992). *Report of the Inquiry into London's Health Service, Medical Education and Research*. London: HMSO.

Townsend, P., Davidson, N. and Whitehead, M. (1988). *Inequalities in Health*. London: Penguin.

Van Weel, C. (1994). Teamwork. *The Lancet*, 344, 1276–9.

Waine, C. (1992). First division united. *Health Service Journal*, 102 (5293), 23.

Walley, T., Wilson, R. and Bligh, J. (1995). Current prescribing in primary care in the UK. *PharmacoEconomics*, 7, 320–31.

Watkin, B. (1978). *The National Health Service: The First Phase*. London: Allen and Unwin.

Wilding, P. (1982). *Professional Power and Social Welfare*. London: Routledge and Kegan Paul.

Wilson, R.P.H., Hatcher, J., Barton, S. and Walley, T. (1996). Influence of practice characteristics on prescribing in fundholding and non-fundholding general practices: an observational study. *British Medical Journal*, 313, 595–9.

Younghusband, Eileen (1978). *Social Work in Britain: 1950–1975*. London: Allen and Unwin.

INDEX

EVALUATING THE NATIONAL HEALTH SERVICE

Martin A. Powell

This is a fresh and innovative study of the National Health Service. Drawing on his unusually wide research experience relating to British health care from the 1930s to the present, Martin Powell avoids the well-worn path by concentrating on the problematic area of evaluation. He demonstrates that balanced assessment of the NHS has been impeded by political correctness and rhetoric to such an extent that it is extremely difficult to arrive at objectively firm conclusions about the record of health service past or present.

In this ambitious, astute and indeed audacious study, Dr Powell penetrates the fog of obfuscation, and outlines a conceptual approach likely to yield more certain conclusions in the future.

Charles Webster, official historian of the NHS

- To what extent has the National Health Service achieved its objectives?
- How well does the performance of the National Health Service compare with health care before the NHS and with other countries?
- What impact have the recent reforms had on the National Health Service?

This book provides the first single, comprehensive evaluation of the National Health Service. It draws on original research to examine health care before the NHS, and health care in other countries in order to locate the service in its wider context. In eight, well-structured chapters it traces the changing policies of the NHS, analyses its successes and failures, examines the current situation in the service, and attempts to predict its future direction.

Evaluating the National Health Service is intended for textbook use by students of social policy, health policy and politics. It is also directly relevant to a wide variety of health care professionals both in training and in practice.

Contents
Introduction – Health care before the NHS – The settlement of 1948 – The NHS 1948–96 – Temporal evaluation – Intrinsic evaluation – Extrinsic evaluation – Conclusion – References – Index

240pp   0 335 19530 X (Paperback)   0 335 19531 8 (Hardback)